therapists' guide
to lower back
and pelvic pain

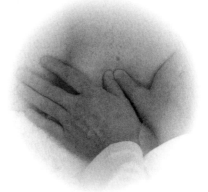

For Churchill Livingstone:

Senior Commissioning Editor: Sarena Wolfaard
Development Editor: Claire Wilson
Project Manager: Elouise Ball
Design: George Ajayi
Illustration Manager: Gillian Richards
Illustrator: Barking Dog Art, Graeme Chambers

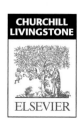

A massage therapists' guide to lower back and pelvic pain

With accompanying DVD

Leon Chaitow ND DO

Registered Osteopathic Practitioner and Senior Lecturer,
University of Westminster, London, UK

Sandy Fritz BS MS

Director, Health Enrichment Center, School of Therapeutic
Massage, Lapeer, MI, USA

Foreword by

Tom Myers

Illustrations by

Graeme Chambers BA(Hons)

Medical Artist

CHURCHILL
LIVINGSTONE

ELSEVIER

EDINBURGH LONDON NEW YORK OXFORD PHILADELPHIA ST LOUIS SYDNEY TORONTO 2007

CHURCHILL
LIVINGSTONE
ELSEVIER

An imprint of Elsevier Ltd

© 2007, Elsevier Ltd. All rights reserved.

First published 2007
Reprinted, 2008

ISBN 9780443102189

British Library Cataloguing in Publication Data
A catalogue record for this book is available from the British Library

Library of Congress Cataloging in Publication Data
A catalog record for this book is available from the Library of Congress

Working together to grow
libraries in developing countries

www.elsevier.com | www.bookaid.org | www.sabre.org

ELSEVIER   BOOK AID International   Sabre Foundation

ELSEVIER   your source for books, journals and multimedia in the health sciences

www.elsevierhealth.com

The publisher's policy is to use **paper manufactured from sustainable forests**

Printed by Uniprint International

Contents

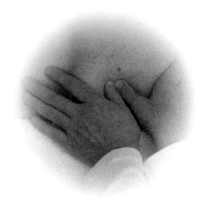

The DVD accompanying this text includes video sequences of all the techniques indicated in the text by the icon. To look at the video for a given technique, click on the relevant icon in the contents list on the DVD. The DVD is designed to be used in conjunction with the text and not as a stand-alone product.

Foreword

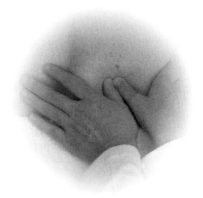

Given the wide range and prodigious output of both Dr Leon Chaitow and Dr Sandy Fritz, it is no surprise that a book that combines their efforts should be well researched, comprehensively presented and generally a treat to read and use. Low Back and Pelvic Pain is a timely subject, and the authors' approach lends itself to contemporary competently trained massage therapists.

Modern medicine is so intricate (and the system for delivering it is so distressed) that both orthopedists and physiotherapists have migrated toward more complex care, aimed at the many simultaneously serious and mysterious pathologic and injury conditions associated with back and pelvic pain. This leaves a large area of non-specific back pain, what could be called sub-clinical pain, which fails to meet the threshold for specified care within the medical system, but is nevertheless somewhere between bothersome and debilitating to the patient. Into this gap steps today's well-trained massage therapist, and he or she will be well advised to come armed with this book.

Our very human process of achieving upright standing – always a precarious balance of the segmented tent pole of our spine swaying above the two small tripods of our feet, with the pelvis arbitrating both stability and mobility between the two – is further challenged these days by the amount of sitting we do before computers and in cars. The original 'thousand ills the flesh is heir to' are further augmented by poor nutritional support and 'one-size fits all' exercise systems that can put significant strain into low back and pelvic tissues.

Easing the resulting strain patterns is well within the purview and skill level of the well-versed, sensitive, observant and curious massage therapist. What has been missing is a resource to guide one through the bewildering range of alternative treatments in light of new and traditional research findings. The book in your hand is just such a map of the current state-of-play for getting such non-specific sufferers out of trouble.

The process begins with the act of 'triage' – determining which cases are appropriate to the massage or manual therapist, versus those that are beyond that level of skill. Today's massage therapist can often be the first health professional who sees the back pain patient (where formerly they might have gone to their GP first). Such increased responsibility must be met with increased assessment skill to separate out those who need advanced care – the signs for which are detailed in this book with clear cautionary 'flags'.

Spinal pathologies and radiculopathies are best addressed with the aid of sophisticated imaging tools and medical procedures, (often supplemented, we hope, with good manual therapy). But there remain a host of less complicated conditions – some temporary, some chronic - resulting from misuse, over-use, chronic structural abuse, parasitic patterns of recruitment, or simple lack of appropriate muscle tonus. These conditions often get better over time by themselves, but massage and movement techniques have been shown to help shorten recovery time, as well as blocking the road to re-injury through preventive movement education.

We could add 'recovery from surgery or other trauma' to this list, since – and while this may not be universally true, it is accurate in many cases indeed – our current medical system allocates inadequate resources, especially that of time, to integrated recovery after medical intervention.

These non-specific pains and integrative rehabilitation patients do not always require the complexities of modern medical care, especially in the hands of these two experienced experts to guide the assessment and treatment of these conditions. Massage, trigger point work, myofascial release, positional release, joint mobilization, recruitment repatterning and stabilization training can all serve to put such clients back on their feet shortly, efficiently, and with less financial outlay all around.

Once this triage is completed, the authors move smoothly into the assessment of the pain, it's sources, and it's connections, mainly using palpatory assessments of muscles, movements (including breathing), and reflex points. A wide array of assessments, tests and treatment methods are presented – with a clear sequence of indicating signs, intents for outcome, cautions and comprehensive techniques combining many approaches for easing pelvic and low back pain syndromes.

In Chapter 7, these techniques are brought together in a series of strategies for using massage and manipulation for restoring full, integrated function. Well illustrated, this section ranges more widely than just the lower torso, to take in the full body, all of which can sometimes be involved in pelvic or lumbar pain through fascial, functional or reflexive connections. In Chapters 8 and 9, the authors explore preventive training and exercise for restoring balance and preventing re-injury.

Every procedure in this volume is backed up with the relevant research references, linking the practitioner with the source material for why the protocol is included, and providing doctors and physiotherapists with sound reasoning for why such approaches work on a scientific and clinical level (and are thus suitable for referral). As such, this book represents a significant step forward in bringing together the intuitive arts of the manual therapist with the scientific backing required by outcomes-based clinical practice.

Use this book for all it is worth – to deepen your practical and theoretical grasp of why non-specific low back and pelvic pain occurs and (more to the point) why it persists, to expand your therapeutic approaches when your own 'library' of manual therapy does not seem to be doing the trick. Finally, 'seal the deal' by helping your patients prevent recurrence and build the strength necessary to a pain free functional life.

Welcome to this new guide to the complex foundation of the human body.

Tom Myers
Walpole Maine USA

Chapter 1

The 'triage'

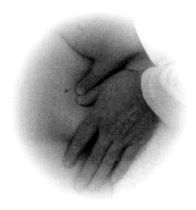

INTRODUCTION

The term 'triage' derives from battlefield settings where wounded soldiers were divided (by the senior physician) into three categories: those with serious injuries who were likely to recover with appropriate attention, and who therefore received primary attention; those with minor wounds whose condition allowed for delay in their receiving treatment; and those whose injuries were so severe that recovery was unlikely and who therefore received only limited attention in the pressured environment of battle.

There is general agreement that low back pain falls into three broad categories, and it is the third on this list that this book will focus on.

Back pain can result from:

1 Serious spinal pathology (or non-spinal pathology that refers to the spine)
2 Nerve root pain (radicular pain)
3 Non-specific causes.

This chapter is devoted to an overview of non-specific back pain, the cause of well over 90% of cases (Deyo & Weinstein 2001).

In Chapter 2, there is a discussion of the main causes and characteristics of back pain that results from the specific causes that we will *not* be focusing on. This is because it is important that you have a basic understanding of the causes and symptoms associated with back pain where serious pathology or nerve root problems (such as a herniated disc) are the causes, even if you are not going to treat those conditions.

Additionally, Chapter 2 will have information regarding a range of health problems that produce symptoms that mimic, or masquerade as, back pain – the so-called *impostor* symptoms.

Once it is established that a person's back pain derives from non-pathological, non-specific, musculo-skeletal causes, it is helpful to establish just what degree of pain the patient is experiencing, and what areas are involved. Methods used to establish pain levels, and the questions that need answering regarding this, are discussed in Chapter 3.

NON-SPECIFIC BACK PAIN

The type of back pain that we are considering in this chapter is the most common form, which commonly has no obvious cause, and usually has no obvious pathology connected to it.

This sort of back pain *is not* directly linked to conditions such as arthritis, a tumour, osteoporosis, ankylosing spondylitis, hypermobility, a fracture, inflammation, nerve compression or cord compression.

Although all of these conditions can cause pain in the back (acute or chronic), so can 'non-specific' factors.

- Often the patient who presents with 'common non-specific backache' is otherwise well. The symptoms usually vary with activity, and this suggests that biomechanical factors are the main aggravating features (Waddell 1998)
- In contrast to non-mechanical backache, where symptoms are often continuous and unremitting, non-specific forms are usually variable, are relieved by rest, and by particular positions and movements (such as stretching). It is therefore very important that you ask your patient specifically: 'Is your pain constant, or does it vary?' If the back pain varies you need to discover what circumstances seem to bring it on or aggravate it
- It is important to remember that 'uncomplicated' does not mean that the pain is a minor feature. The pain of uncomplicated backache may be extreme, often spreading to the buttocks and thighs
- Contributing causes, leading to non-specific back pain, may include poor posture, over-use, decon-ditioning (poor muscle tone, lack of exercise), chills, trigger point activity, and/or other factors, many of which the person with the back pain may be able to control or modify.

Many of these factors will be expanded upon in Chapter 4, which concentrates on the connection between how the body is used, how it is 'cared for', and back pain. Management of back pain will be seen – in that chapter and others – to have a great deal to do with self-management/self-care, with the therapist offering advice and treatment, but with the 'owner' of the back having primary responsibility for its rehabili-tation and maintenance.

Making sure there is a correct diagnosis

It is important for you to try to identify and under-stand what may be causing or aggravating your patient's back pain, so that you can offer appropriate advice as to how to improve the condition through self-directed management and rehabilitation strategies.

As will be outlined later in this chapter (and expanded upon in Chapter 2), there are numerous 'impostor' (or 'masquerader') symptoms that it is necessary to be aware of, because a patient's back pain may at times be the result of serious health problems.

If there is any doubt at all as to what is causing the back pain, a clear diagnosis should be obtained from an appropriately licensed practitioner (Grieve 1994). This does not mean that massage and manual treat-ment, together with appropriate exercise and move-ment, cannot help back pain that *is* linked to serious pathology, but the main focus of this book is not towards such conditions because, as a rule, the more serious causes of back pain require medical or specialist (e.g. osteopathic, chiropractic, physical therapy) management (Eisenberg et al 1998).

Our interest, in this book, is on the huge majority (97%) of back pain problems, that result from mechanical causes such as a strain, or an awkward movement, or being in a static stressful position for too long; or which develop when a combination of minor stresses occur together (Deyo & Weinstein 2001).

As for the other 3%, if any 'red' or 'yellow' flags emerge when you are taking the case history of the patient with back pain you should suggest a referral to a licensed practitioner whose scope of practice allows the making of an accurate diagnosis. These 'flags' are touched on later in the chapter, and are explained and discussed more fully in Chapter 2. In such cases, the patient should be told that once a diagnosis has been made, you will be more than happy to offer appro-priate massage therapy to help ease the symptoms, and hopefully to facilitate recovery, but that for you to do so *before* a diagnosis is available would be inappro-priate and unethical.

If you ensure a diagnosis in cases where the cause of the back pain is unknown, your ethical, legal and professional position will be reinforced.

COST AND RANGE OF BACK PAIN

The human and economic cost of back pain is simply enormous:

- Lower-back (and neck) pain are the two largest causes of time off work (Andersson 1997)
- Back pain is the most frequent reason that causes people to consult with complementary or alter-native therapists and practitioners (Grieve 1994)

- and back pain is the second most common reason for a visit to the MD (Deyo & Weinstein 2001)
- and back pain is the cause of excessive use of radiological imaging and surgery
- and back pain is also the most expensive work-related cause of disability (Grieve 1994)
- Four out of five people suffer back pain at least once (Bigos et al 1994), and 65 million adults are affected by back pain in the USA each year (Deyo & Weinstein 2001)
- Andersson (1997) reports that, in industrialized countries, 70% of people experience acute low back pain at least once, and that in any given year, between 15 and 45% will do so.

Just how costly is back pain?

Luo et al (2004) estimate the cost to the US economy as being more than US$90 billion annually, broken down as follows:

- US$27.9bn in-patient care
- US$23.6bn office visits
- US$14.1bn prescription drugs
- US$11.9bn outpatient services (occupational therapy, physical therapy, etc.)
- US$2.7bn emergency room visits
- US$10.5bn miscellaneous.

When the cost of social security payments, and loss of productivity, are also taken into account, Eisenberg (2004) goes far beyond these obvious costs, and suggests that the total cost of back pain to the US economy is in excess of US$*190 billion per year* – accounting for around 1% of the gross national product of the USA.

MASSAGE AND BACK PAIN

Back pain can be seen to be a major problem. It represents a burden for the patient, the family, and increasingly, for the economy of industrialized countries. Within that huge problem, massage, along with complementary soft tissue and joint treatment methods, have been shown to offer safe and effective care to assist in recovery and rehabilitation (Ernst 2000).

Cherkin et al (2003) in their research review have compared massage with manipulation and acupuncture in treating back pain, and have found massage to be safe, and to be superior in both effectiveness and cost-effectiveness to the other methods:

> Initial studies have found massage to be effective for persistent back pain. Spinal manipulation has small clinical benefits that are equivalent to those of other commonly used therapies. The effectiveness of acupuncture remains unclear. All of these

treatments seem to be relatively safe. Preliminary evidence suggests that massage, but not acupuncture or spinal manipulation, may reduce the costs of care after an initial course of therapy.

WHAT ARE THE VARIOUS ELEMENTS THAT LEAD TO BACK PAIN?

Back pain can have various underlying biomechanical causes, including injury to the muscles or ligaments in the back, compression of the nerves in the spine, and damage to the discs that cushion the vertebrae, or the facets of the spinal joints. Whatever the contributory factors, and immediate triggers, that lead to back pain, it is safe to say that the real 'cause' is almost always a failure of adaptation (Selye 1956). To understand adaptation, see Box 1.1.

Whether sprains and strains are acute, involving sudden trauma, or are the result of gradual 'wear and tear', these minor traumas involve a failure of the structures of the area to cope with the demands being imposed on them. Such failure often leads to tissue damage (microtrauma – or more serious trauma) inflammation, nerve irritation, and ultimately pain.

The causes of back pain can usually be shown to involve a variable set of ingredients because factors such as age, inherited features (take for example hyper-mobility or limbs of unequal length, etc.), general nutritional and fitness (aerobic) status, as well as the nature, degree, frequency and duration of the 'load' being dealt with/adapted to, all enter into the equation. It is logical to assume that a young, fit, balanced set of muscles and joints will almost always manage a lifting task better than an elderly, unfit, unbalanced set of muscles and joints (Paris 1997).

'CAUSES' OF NON-SPECIFIC BACK PAIN

A number of different factors and features, all of which can contribute to or help maintain back pain are summarized below. The symptoms and effects of those activities that are within the influence of massage therapists will be expanded on in later chapters.

The most commonly reported 'causes' of low back pain are (Andersson 1997):

- Heavy physical work
- Bending
- Twisting
- Lifting
- Pulling and pushing
- Repetitive work patterns
- Static postures
- Vibrations.

Box 1.1   Adaptation

Adaptation represents the story of the contest between the 'load' and the tissues handling the load.

Tissues adapt to the load imposed on them. Think of athletic or weight training as easy examples. To run the marathon, or perform the high jump, or any other specialized task or activity (gardening, working on a production line, painting ceilings, etc.) particular muscles and joints have repetitive demands imposed on them.

After an initial acute alarm phase of the local adaptation syndromes (LAS) or general adaptation syndromes (GAS), when stiffness and soreness may be experienced, the tissues start to adapt, and no longer react with stiffness and soreness. This is the adaptation phase of LAS (involving a local area, such the shoulders or knees) or GAS (involving the whole person), which continues until the load (the stress demands) reduces, or the tissues themselves can no longer adapt (like a piece of tired elastic), at which time the 'breakdown', or 'exhaustion' phase of LAS or GAS (Fig. 1.1) starts and symptoms of pain and dysfunction become apparent (Selye 1956).

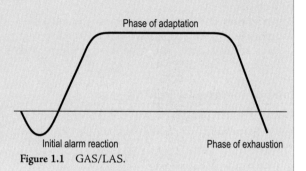

Figure 1.1   GAS/LAS.

Most of these causes, or triggers, of the onset of back pain involve poor use of the body. It is relatively easy to learn better ways of bending, lifting, moving and carrying, and appropriately illustrated educational hand-out notes should be supplied to patients, along with demonstrations of better use patterns (Fig. 1.2).

The close environment and back pain

It is also useful to ask yourself what features of the person's close environment might be contributing to the back pain.

Ill-fitting and poorly designed shoes (platforms, stiletto heels, etc.; Fig. 1.3) as well as stress-inducing chairs, and cramped or distorting driving or working positions, are just some factors that might fit into the category of 'close environment' stressors, in any given case.

Psychosocial contributions to back pain

The most common psychosocial risk factors contributing to back pain have been listed (Hoogendoorn et al 2000, Linton 2000) as being:

- Stress: feelings of being overwhelmed by the demands of life, time pressures, etc.

- Distress: a combination of feelings of helplessness and unhappiness
- Anxiety: an exaggerated level of concern and fear, possibly involving 'catastrophizing', where the future is seen as bleak, and almost always involving altered (usually 'upper chest') breathing patterns, that contribute to lowered pain threshold and altered muscle tone (Chaitow et al 2002, Nixon & Andrews 1996)
- Depression: a profound unhappiness and sense of existence being pointless
- Cognitive dysfunction: a misunderstanding and/or misinterpretation of facts
- Pain behavior: avoiding normal everyday activities that it is feared *might* aggravate the back pain problem
- Job dissatisfaction: blaming the job for the back problem, or simply unhappiness in the work situation
- Mental stress at work or in the home: inter-personal tensions, time (or other) pressures that make working and/or home environments unsatisfying or actively unpleasant.

Remedies for many of these psychosocial factors are to be found through patient education, stress management, counseling and cognitive behavioral therapy (Moore et al 2000).

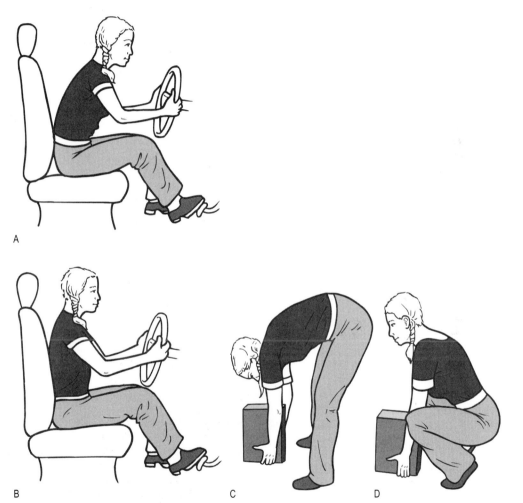

A

B

C

D

Figure 1.2   Bad and better use patterns. Driving: (A) incorrect and (B) correct. Lifting: (C) incorrect and (D) correct. (From Chaitow and Fritz 2006.)

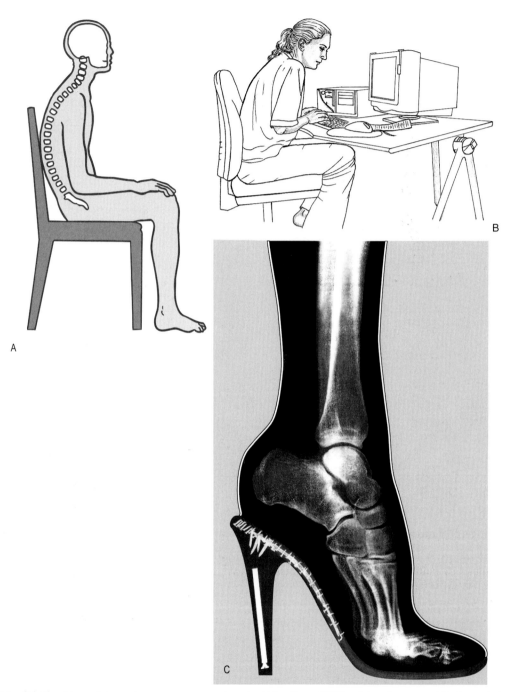

Figure 1.3 (A) The right angled seated posture encourages slumping (After Cranz 2000) and, in order to see while slumped, the head rotates back in relation to the top vertebra, exerting a downward pressure on the spine. (B) (From Wilson 2001.) (C) Footwear has a significant impact on the foot, the extreme of which is illustrated in the high-heel shoe. Distortions of the foot will be reflected into the rest of the body with significant postural and structural implications. (From Chaitow and DeLany 2002.)

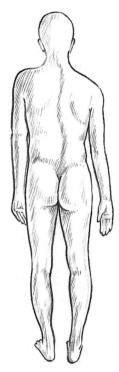

Figure 1.4   Structural imbalance resulting in scoliotic pattern when standing occurs as a result of short (right) leg. An adequate heel lift placed under the short leg should result in straightening of the spine, unless the spine is rigidly fixed (after Travell & Simons 1992). (From Chaitow and DeLany 2002.)

In-born, congenital and acquired features and back pain

A part of the back pain story may relate to stresses arising from features such as:

- one leg being shorter/longer than the other (Fig. 1.4)
- one side of the pelvis being smaller than the other
- the upper arms being unusually short causing the person to lean sideways when seated in an arm chair
- unusual foot structures (such as Morton's syndrome) (Frey 1994)
- unusual degrees of hypermobility (laxness) of the connective tissue (Keer & Grahame 2003)
- being extremely overweight.

THE BIOMECHANICS OF BACK PAIN: THE MOTOR SYSTEM

To understand the background to a great deal of non-specific back pain, you need to be familiar with the system that offers stability to joints and facilitates their ability to be moved by attaching muscles: the motor system.

Panjabi (1992) has shown that the motor system is made up of three inter-related elements:

1 *The central nervous subsystem (control)*: the central nervous system and brain respond to proprioceptive input (messages that inform the brain about the status of the tissues being reported on: are the tissues tense? are they moving? if so how fast? is anything restricting them? etc.). Messages arrive from the tens of thousands of reporting stations throughout the body and, based on the information received, decisions are made (to move, change position, stand, walk, etc.). Instructions are given to the muscles to perform actions to increase or decrease tone, or to actively contract in order to create movement of a joint or limb, or area. Some actions are automatic (reflex) and some are a mixture of responses to proprioceptive input, and deliberate choices about activity (to stand up, sit down, walk, to scratch, etc.).

2 *The osteoligamentous subsystem (passive)*: this is the system that binds and supports the joints, offering stability to the movement and stabilizing the functions of joints. These activities are outside of voluntary control. If there is relative laxity (hypermobility, looseness) of structures such as the ligaments, function – such as movement – will be less efficiently and safely achieved. Some aspects of this subsystem are osseous, for example the form and shape of the bones of the pelvis that meet at the sacroiliac joint can be so configured as to offer a solid base on which the pelvis can work. However, the structures can be poorly matched, offering relatively poor 'form' closure, leading to an unstable joint (Lee 1999). This will be explained in Chapter 5, which looks at the pelvis and its contribution to back stability, or back problems.

3 *The muscle subsystem (active)*: the status and interrelationship between muscles that perform stabilizing (postural-type 1) tasks, and those that perform active (phasic-type 2) movement functions, decides how efficiently, and with what degree of fine-control, movement occurs.

Anything that interferes with any aspect of these three features of normal motor control, may contribute to dysfunction and pain (Lewit 1999). See Box 1.2 on the topic of postural and phasic muscles.

Box 1.2 Postural and phasic muscles

There are basically two types of muscles in the body: those that have as their main task stabilization, and those that have as their main task movement (Engel 1986, Woo et al 1987).

These are known as:

- *Postural* (also known as Type I, or 'slow twitch red') and
- *Phasic* (also known as Type II, or 'fast twitch white') (Janda 1982).

It is not within the scope of this book to provide detailed physiological descriptions of the differences between these muscle types, but it is important to know that:

- All muscles contain both types of fiber (Type I and Type II) but that the predominance of one type over the other determines the nature of that particular muscle
- Postural muscles have very low stores of energy-supplying glycogen but carry high concentrations of myoglobulin and mitochondria. These fibers fatigue slowly and are mainly involved in postural and stabilizing tasks, and when stressed (overused, underused, traumatized), tend to shorten over time
- Phasic muscles contract more rapidly than postural fibers, have variable but reduced resistance to fatigue, and when stressed (overused, underused, traumatized) tend to weaken, and sometimes to lengthen over time
- There are a variety of Type II fibers
- Evidence exists of the potential for adaptability of muscle fibers. For example, slow-twitch can convert to fast-twitch and vice versa, depending upon the patterns of use to which they are put, and the stresses they endure (Lin 1994). An example of this involves the scalene muscles which Lewit (1999) confirms can be classified as either a postural or a phasic muscle. If stressed (as in asthma), the scalenes will change from a phasic to become a postural muscle
- Trigger points can form in either type of muscles in response to local situations of stress.

Summary

Postural muscles: Those muscles that shorten in response to dysfunction (Fig. 1.5), which include:

- Trapezius (upper), sternocleidomastoid, levator scapulae and upper aspects of pectoralis major, in the upper trunk; and the flexors of the arms
- Quadratus lumborum, erector spinae, oblique abdominals and iliopsoas, in the lower trunk
- Tensor fascia lata, rectus femoris, biceps femoris, adductors (longus brevis and magnus) piriformis, hamstrings, semitendinosus, in the pelvic and lower extremity region.

Phasic muscles: Those muscles that weaken in response to dysfunction (i.e. are inhibited), which include:

- The paravertebral muscles (not erector spinae), scalenes (see above), the extensors of the upper extremity, the abdominal aspects of pectoralis major; middle and inferior aspects of trapezius; the rhomboids, serratus anterior, rectus abdominus; the internal and external obliques, gluteals, the peroneal muscles and the extensors of the arms.

A useful chart (below) can be used to chart changes (shortening) in the main postural muscles.

Postural muscle assessment sequence

NAME: _____

Key: E Equal (circle both if both are short)
L & R are circled if left or right are short
Spinal abbreviations – indicating areas of *flatness* during flexion, and therefore reduced ability to flex – suggesting shortened erector spinae:

LL	low lumbar	LDJ	lumbo-dorsal junction
LT	low-thoracic	MT	mid-thoracic
UT	upper thoracic		

01	Gastrocnemius		E	L	R	
02	Soleus		E	L	R	
03	Medial hamstrings		E	L	R	
04	Short adductors		E	L	R	
05	Rectus femoris		E	L	R	
06	Psoas		E	L	R	
07	Hamstrings					
	a upper fires		E	L	R	
	b lower fires		E	L	R	
08	Tensor fascia lata		E	L	R	
09	Piriformis		E	L	R	
10	Quadratus lumborum		E	L	R	
11	Pectoralis major		E	L	R	
12	Latissimus dorsi		E	L	R	
13	Upper trapezius		E	L	R	
14	Scalenes		E	L	R	
15	Sternocleidomastoid		E	L	R	
16	Levator scapulae		E	L	R	
17	Infraspinatus		E	L	R	
18	Subscapularis		E	L	R	
19	Supraspinatus		E	L	R	
20	Flexors of the arm		E	L	R	
21	Spinal flattening					
	a seated legs straight	LL	LDJ	LT	MT	UT
	b seated legs flexed	LL	LDJ	LT	MT	UT
	c Cervical spine extensors short?	Yes	No			

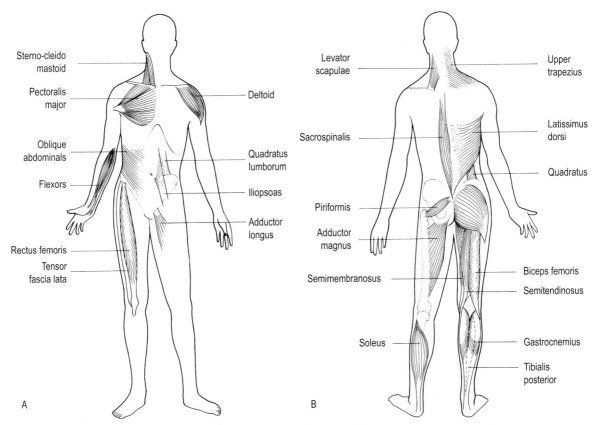

Figure 1.5   (A) The major postural muscles of the anterior aspect of the body. (B) The major postural muscles of the posterior aspect of the body.

STABILITY

To continue with the sacroiliac example, if the muscles that attach to the pelvis are unbalanced, some being too tight, others too weak (lax), for whatever reason, 'force' closure of the SI joint may be compromised, with back and pelvic pain resulting. Force closure is explained in Chapter 5, along with 'form' closure issues.

The key muscles that determine the stability and functionality of the back and the pelvis are (Van Tulder et al 2004):

- Rectus abdominis
- External obliques
- Internal obliques
- Latissimus dorsi
- Pars lumborum
- Iliocostalis lumborum
- Longissimus thoracis
- Quadratus lumborum
- Multifidus
- Transversus abdominis

- Psoas
- Piriformis
- Gluteus maximus and medius.

ASSESSING FOR MUSCLE STRENGTH, STAMINA, LENGTH, COORDINATION AND TRIGGER POINTS

Ideally, depending on the region affected by, or contributing to the patient's reported back pain, it is helpful to know the current status of the associated muscles:

- Do the patient's phasic (Type 2) muscles have adequate strength to perform their movement tasks? This can be tested by using 'strength tests' and where appropriate exercise to facilitate strength can be advised (see Ch. 3)
- Do the patient's postural (Type 1) muscles have adequate stamina to perform their stabilizing tasks? Simple tests can help identify muscles that need to be trained to regain their stamina (see Ch. 3)

- Have the patient's Type 1 muscles shortened (that is, is there any loss of range of motion)? Testing for length (shortness or over-lengthened) can be performed to identify those in need of appropriate treatment (see Ch. 3)
- Is there good coordination between those muscles that cooperate and support each other (synergists) in particular movements? Testing movements (such as hip abduction) to see whether muscle firing sequences are coordinated are described in Chapter 4
- Are there active or latent trigger points in any of the key muscles relating to the painful area? Palpation and treatment methods are described throughout the rest of the book
- Does stretching of any of the local muscles cause discomfort or pain? If so, this may indicate the presence of active trigger points in the muscle
- Are local reflexes normal? Testing reflexes helps establish whether nerve function is over- or under-active (see Ch. 3).

In Chapters 4, 5, 6 and 7 we will look at massage and other manual therapy methods that will allow you to palpate, assess and treat dysfunctional aspects of these muscles.

SOME OF THE MANY CONTRIBUTORY FEATURES OF NON-SPECIFIC BACK PAIN

As will become clear, when we have looked at the various parts of this complicated picture, there are numerous features and factors that can interfere with the ability of muscles to perform their support and movement tasks (motor control), resulting in back pain, including:

- trigger point activity (Simons et al 1999)
- deconditioning/disuse (the opposite of being aerobically conditioned) (Nixon & Andrews 1996)
- disturbed balance (Winters & Crago 2000)
- disturbed information gathering (proprioceptive input, including visual and auditory signals)
- hypermobility (Muller et al 2003)
- hyperventilation (Lum 1987)
- anxiety and other emotional states (Vlaeyen & Crombez 1999)
- poor nutrition (Brostoff 1992)
- inflammation (Handwerker & Reeh 1991)
- endocrine disturbances (such as underactive thyroid) (Lowe & Honeyman-Lowe 1998)
- poor posture (physiological 'misuse') (Lewit 1999)
- overuse and trauma (abuse).

McGill (2004) summarizes this as follows: 'The muscular and motor system must satisfy the requirements to sustain postures, create movements, brace against sudden motion or unexpected forces, build pressure, and assist challenged breathing, all the while ensuring sufficient stability'. The most important of these potential contributory factors will be discussed in Chapter 4.

CAUTIONS: RED AND YELLOW FLAGS

Red flags are signs that may be present, alongside acute back pain, that suggest that possibly serious factors – often pathological – are operating. These are described in more detail in Chapter 2.

Unlike the possibly pathological signs that the red flags represent, yellow flags are described as suggesting psychosocial factors that 'increase the risk of developing, or perpetuating chronic pain and long-term disability. These are also more fully explained in Chapter 2 (RCGP 1999, Van Tulder et al 2004).

Recognizing yellow flag signs should alert you to the need for appropriate counseling or psychotherapy, or at the very least what is known as cognitive behavior therapy (see Box 1.3).

Avoid bed rest unless essential

Once serious pathology has been ruled out, various modalities may help in treating back pain, including massage, deactivation of local trigger points (that can be responsible for much neck and back pain), manipulation, stretching, ultrasound, hydrotherapy and exercise. But whatever else is done, in most cases of back pain, there is a great deal of evidence that it is important *not* to take to bed (unless it is absolutely necessary, as in some acute disc herniation situations).

A review of many studies concluded that bed rest:

- has no positive effect for back pain
- may have slightly harmful effects (Hagen et al 2000).

Improved habits of use

In the long term, learning new ways of standing, walking, sitting and working can be very important in preventing repeated episodes of back and neck problems. These issues will be discussed further in Chapters 8 and 9 (Hides et al 2001). Sometimes quite simple changes can reduce the chance of recurrence:

Box 1.3   Cognitive behavioral therapy

Modern pain management programs commonly use cognitive behavioral therapy (CBT) to reverse, or change, 'illness behavior'.

If an activity is painful, stopping that activity may relieve the pain in the short term but this may condition the person to avoidance of pain by doing less and less, leading to a belief that pain is an indication of increased harm. This leads to deconditioning, and usually does little to improve the pain problem.

If the person with back pain is observed by a family member, or friend, to be having difficulty doing something, that person might perform the task instead. This can 'teach' the person in pain to avoid particular activities, because it becomes preferable to let someone else perform the task.

These examples of changed behavior in response to pain are known as *operant conditioning* and CBT methods are designed to reverse these negative behavior patterns (Wall & Melzack 1989).

The message that 'hurt does not necessarily mean harm' is one of the important lessons the person in pain needs to learn. To achieve this, CBT methods (Bradley 1996, Turk et al 1983) focus on:

- *Education*: learning about the painful condition. What it is and what it is not
- *Skills training*: learning to use the body more efficiently and less stressfully
- *Skills rehearsal and feedback*: learning to become familiar with and to apply these new skills

- *Generalization of skills taught to use in everyday situations, and in novel situations*: learning how to use new skills in a variety of settings, some unexpected.

The objectives of interdisciplinary pain management and CBT are to:

- Assist patients to modify their belief that their problems are unmanageable and beyond their control
- Inform patients about their condition
- Assist patients to move from a passive to an active role in the management of their condition
- Enable patients to become active problem-solvers to help them cope with their pain through the development of effective ways of responding to pain, emotion and the environment
- Help patients to monitor thought, emotions and behaviors, and identify how these are influenced by internal and external events
- Give patients a feeling of competence in the execution of positive strategies in the management of their condition
- Help patients to develop a positive attitude to exercise and personal health management
- Help patients to develop a program of paced activity to reduce the effects of physical deconditioning
- Assist patients to develop coping strategies that can be developed, once contact with the pain management team, or healthcare provider, has ended.

- Simply wearing cushioned insoles can reduce stress on spinal tissues, reducing the chances of back pain (Paris 1997)
- Additionally, it is known that one of the most vulnerable times for the low back is early morning, soon after getting up from the bed, particularly when bending forward (putting on socks, for example) (Liebenson 2000, Snook et al 1998).

Avoidance of such 'high risk' activities, early in the morning, or after sitting for any length of time, is helpful in both injury, and re-injury, prevention. Research has shown that avoiding early morning bending helps recovery from acute low back pain (Snook et al 2002).

TREATMENT

The fact is that most backaches recover in between 3 and 6 weeks, with or without treatment, although there is evidence that massage and manipulation (such as is used in chiropractic and osteopathy) help the period of recovery to be more comfortable (Meade et al 1995).

In both the short and the long term, whether manipulation is more effective than exercise, and/or re-education, in helping normalize back pain remains controversial, because many research studies seem to contradict each other (Blomberg et al 1992, Triano et al 1995).

A 1997 national survey showed that, apart from visiting a mainstream physician, massage was among the most popular complementary treatments for back pain, alongside acupuncture, herbal remedies and spinal manipulation (Eisenberg et al 1998). This research found that 48% of adults with low back pain used at least one complementary therapy.

The most commonly used complementary modalities were:

- chiropractic
- massage therapy
- acupuncture
- mind–body techniques.

How successful are these methods?

If adaptation (see Box 1.1) is the primary cause of back and neck pain, then whatever treatment is offered should achieve one of three things:

1 removal or reduction in the stress load to which the local tissues (or the body as a whole) are adapting
2 improvement in the way(s) the local tissues (or the body as whole) are coping, adapting
3 symptomatic treatment to make the recovery period more comfortable, without adding to the adaptive load.

Sometimes all three elements can be achieved, sometimes only one.

Since healing and recovery is a self-generated function (cuts heal, broken bones mend, etc.), the important element in any treatment choice is that it should be safe, should not add to the load, and should hopefully help recovery to be more rapidly achieved, and if not, at least more comfortably.

Massage seems well able to offer a number of these features, with education and rehabilitation exercises doing the rest in most cases.

Massage

What research has shown
It is important to know that most acute back problems are self-limiting. Around 90% of people with an acute back problem will be better within 6 weeks, whatever treatment they receive (unless it is a form of treatment that makes things worse!).

However, between 2 and 7% of people with an acute back pain problem will develop chronic back pain, and it is this category that is most worrying because around 80% of work absenteeism is the result of chronic back pain (Andersson 1997).

Back pain is often associated with a complicated dysfunction of the paraspinal and other back muscles (Cooper 1993). It is possible that in many cases, massaging these could help improve or normalize muscular function, and research (Cherkin et al 2001) suggests

this is so. Professor Edzard Ernst (1999) reports that, 'On the European continent, massage has been a routine form of therapy for acute and chronic LBP for many decades' (Westhof & Ernst 1992). A recent survey from Vienna shows that no less than 87% of back pain patients received massage as one form of treatment (Ernst & Fialka 1994). Classical Swedish muscle massage has a long history (Westhof & Ernst 1992) and is associated with various effects that are potentially beneficial in the symptomatic treatment of neck and back pain:

- Massage relaxes the mind as well as the musculature and we have seen ('yellow flags') that in many instances of chronic back pain, emotion and stress are possible key features
- Massage increases the pain threshold, possibly through endorphin release (Ernst & Fialka 1994)
- It can also enhance local blood flow and this could increase the clearance of local biochemical substances that increase pain (Ernst & Fialka 1994).

These known beneficial effects of massage do not however *prove* that massage is helpful in treatment of back pain, but fortunately there are studies that do suggest this (Ernst 1994, Triano et al 1995, Wiesinger et al 1997).

Unfortunately, many research reviews entirely ignore massage as a meaningful therapeutic option (Deyo 1983, Frank 1993, Frymoyer 1988, Nachemson 1985) and some physiotherapy texts do not mention it at all (Frost & Moffett 1992).

Proof of the value of massage in treatment of low back pain
Much research has proved the value of massage in the treatment of low back pain (see, e.g. Bronfort et al 2004, Cherkin et al 2003, Ernst 1999). Cherkin et al (2003) pointed out that: 'Few treatments for back pain are supported by strong scientific evidence. Conventional treatments, although widely used, have had limited success. Dissatisfied patients have, therefore, turned to complementary and alternative medical therapies and providers for care for back pain'.

1 Cherkin et al (2003) conducted a summary of all good research on the subject since 1995, in which different methods were compared in treatment of back and/or neck pain. They found 20 research studies that were of a standard to include in their review, however only three evaluated the benefits of massage. The finding of these studies was that 'massage therapy is both safe and effective for subacute and chronic back pain'. They also found that there was evidence that spinal manipulation produced small clinical benefits that are equivalent

to those of other commonly used therapies, but that the effectiveness of acupuncture remains unclear for these problems. Importantly, they found that there is evidence that massage, but not acupuncture or spinal manipulation, may reduce the costs of care after an initial course of therapy in treatment of back pain.

2 In a straight comparison of massage and acupuncture in treating back pain, Frey (1994) found that those receiving massage used the least medications and that: 'Therapeutic massage was effective for persistent low back pain, apparently providing long-lasting benefits. Traditional Chinese Medical acupuncture was relatively ineffective. Massage might be an effective alternative to conventional medical care for persistent back pain'.

3 Güthlin and Walach (2000) conducted a study of patients with 'non-inflammatory rheumatic pain' (not just back pain) who received either 10 sessions of classical massage or usual medical care for 5 weeks. By the end of this period, both groups had improved similarly, but at the 3-month follow-up, more pain relief had occurred in the massage group.

4 Another review (Furlan et al 2000) of research compared massage with de-tuned laser therapy as the placebo, and with various other physical treatments such as acupuncture or spinal manipulation. The results showed that massage is superior to placebo, relaxation treatment, acupuncture, or self-care education, but that it is inferior to manipulation, shiatsu, or transcutaneous electrical stimulation; and no different from treatment with corsets or exercise in the care of back pain. The authors concluded that massage 'might' be beneficial for subacute and chronic non-specific low back pain.

5 Researchers at the Touch Research Institute, Miami School of Medicine, evaluated the benefits of massage when treating low back pain (Hernandez-Reif et al 2001). They summarized the research outcome as follows: 'Adults with low back pain, with a duration of at least 6 months received two 30-min massage, or relaxation therapy, sessions per week for 5 weeks. Participants receiving massage therapy reported experiencing less pain, depression and anxiety and their sleep improved. They also showed improved trunk flexion performance'.

Thus the evidence from these reviews and studies proves that when massage is compared with other treatment methods such as acupuncture, manipulation, relaxation and ultrasound:

- Massage is at least as helpful in treating back pain as other modalities
- Massage reduces use and therefore costs of medication when treating back pain
- Massage as a treatment of back and neck pain is safe.

CONCLUSION

By avoiding the dangers of inappropriate treatment of red and yellow flag patients, and by adding to the undoubted benefits of massage a number of essential rehabilitation features such as core stability and balance training, as well as potentially useful soft tissue manipulation methods (such as trigger point deactivation, muscle energy, positional release, and myofascial release techniques), as described in later chapters, the results should be even better.

KEY POINTS

- Back pain can be associated with neurological or pathological causes, but can also (the vast majority) be 'non-specific'
- A failure to adapt to biomechanical (and/or psychological) adaptive demands seems to lie behind most non-specific back and neck pain problems
- Most back pain gets better with or without treatment, but appropriate treatment can speed the process, and add to comfort during recovery
- Massage can potentially be of great value in treating all forms of back and neck pain, but it is most valuable in treating non-specific forms
- Red and yellow flags should be looked for to alert you to referral for a diagnosis if you are not absolutely sure that a patient's back pain is 'non-specific'
- Faulty motor control is a key cause of back pain
- Faulty motor control can derive from overuse, misuse, abuse and disuse
- Faulty motor control can derive from the influence of myofascial trigger points
- Restoration of motor control commonly requires exercise and/or postural, respiratory and/or balance rehabilitation
- Bed-rest is almost never of value for non-specific back pain
- 'Pain behavior' is a very real danger and should be avoided ('hurt does not necessarily mean harm')
- There are ideal care-sequences that should be incorporated wherever possible, in order to ensure that there are no gaps in the care offered to patients.

References

Andersson G B J 1997 The epidemiology of spinal disorders. In: Frymoyer J W (ed.) The adult spine: principles and practice, 2nd edn. Raven Press, New York, p 93–141

Bigos S, Bowyer O, Braen G et al 1994 Acute low back problems in adults. Guideline No. 14, publication No. 95-0643. Public Health Service, US Department of Health and Human Services, Rockville

Blomberg S, Svardsudd K, Mildenberger F 1992 Controlled multicenter trial of manual therapy in low back pain: initial status, sick leave and pain score during follow up. Orthopaedic Medicine 16:1

Bradley L A 1996 Cognitive therapy for chronic pain. In: Gatchel R J, Turk D C (eds) Psychological approaches to pain management. Guildford Press, New York, p 131–147

Bronfort G, Haas M, Evan R 2004 Efficacy of spinal manipulation and mobilization for low back pain and neck pain: a systematic review and best evidence synthesis. The Spine Journal 4:335–356

Brostoff J 1992 Complete guide to food allergy. Bloomsbury, London

Chaitow L 2001 Muscle energy techniques, 2nd edn. Churchill Livingstone, Edinburgh

Chaitow L, DeLany J 2002 Clinical applications of neuromuscular technique, Volume 2. Churchill Livingstone, Edinburgh

Chaitow L, Fritz S 2006 A massage therapist's guide to understanding, locating and treating myofascial trigger points. Churchill Livingstone, Edinburgh

Chaitow L, Bradley D, Gilbert C 2002 Multidisciplinary approaches to breathing pattern disorders. Churchill Livingstone, Edinburgh

Cherkin D, Eisenberg D, Sherman K et al 2001 Randomized trial comparing traditional Chinese medical acupuncture, therapeutic massage, and self-care education for chronic low back pain. Archives of Internal Medicine 161:1088

Cherkin D, Sherman K, Deyo R et al 2003 A review of the evidence for the effectiveness, safety, and cost of acupuncture, massage therapy, and spinal manipulation for back pain. Annals of Internal Medicine 138:898–906

Cooper R 1993 Understanding paraspinal muscle dysfunction in low back pain a way forward? Annals of Rheumatic Disease 52:413–415

Cranz G 2000 The Alexander Technique in the world of design: posture and the common chair: Part 1: the chair as health hazard. Journal of Bodywork and Movement Therapies 4(2):90–98

Deyo R 1983 Conservative therapy for low back pain distinguishing useful from useless therapy. Journal of the American Medical Association 250:1057–1062

Deyo R, Weinstein J 2001 Low back pain. New England Journal of Medicine 344:363–370

Eisenberg D 2004 Presentation at the International Symposium on the Science of Touch, May 2004, Montreal, Canada

Eisenberg D, David R, Ettner S et al 1998 Trends in alternative medicine use in the United States; 1990–1997. Journal of the American Medical Association 280:1569–1575

Engel A 1986 Skeletal muscle types in myology. McGraw-Hill, New York

Ernst E 1994 Mechanotherapie. WMW 20:504–508

Ernst E 1999 Massage therapy for low back pain: a systematic review. Journal of Pain and Symptom Management 17:65–69

Ernst E 2000 Complementary and alternative medicine in rheumatology. Baillière's Best Practice and Research in Clinical Rheumatology 14:731–749

Ernst E, Fialka V 1994 The clinical effectiveness of massage therapy – a critical review. Forsch Komplementärmed 1:226–232

Forbes St C R, Clair W, Jayson M 1992 Radiographic demonstration of paraspinal muscle wasting in patients with chronic low back pain. British Journal of Rheumatology 31:389–394

Frank A 1993 Low back pain. British Medical Journal 306:901–909

Frey C 1994 Current practice in foot and ankle surgery. McGraw-Hill, New York

Frost H, Moffett J 1992 Physiotherapy management of chronic low back pain. Physiotherapy 78:751–754

Frymoyer J 1988 Back pain and sciatica. New England Journal of Medicine 318:291–300

Furlan A D, Brosseau L, Welch V et al 2000 Massage for low back pain. Cochrane Database System Review CD001929

Grieve G 1994 The masqueraders. In: Boyling J D, Palastanga N (eds) Grieve's modern manual therapy, 2nd edn. Churchill Livingstone, Edinburgh

Güthlin C, Walach H 2000 Die Wirksamkeit der klassichen Massage bei Schmerzpatienten-eine vergleichende Studie. Physikalische Therapie 21:717–722

Hagen K, Hilde G, Jamtvedt G 2000 The Cochrane review of bed rest for acute low back pain and sciatica. Spine 25:2932–2939

Handwerker H, Reeh P 1991 Pain and inflammation. Proceedings of the VIth World Congress on Pain, Pain Research and Clinical Management. Elsevier, Amsterdam, p 59–70

Hernandez-Reif M, Field T, Krasnegor J 2001 Lower back pain is reduced and range of motion increased after massage therapy. International Journal of Neuroscience 106:131–145

Hides J, Jull G, Richardson C 2001 Long term effects of specific stabilising exercises for first episode low back pain. Spine 26:243–248

Hoogendoorn W et al 2000 Systematic review of psychosocial factors as risk factors for back pain. Spine 25:2114–2125

Janda V 1982 Introduction to functional pathology of the motor system. Proceedings of VIIth Commonwealth and International Conference on Sport. Physiotherapy in Sport 3:39

Keer R, Grahame R 2003 Hypermobility syndrome. Butterworth Heinemann, Edinburgh

Lee D 1999 The pelvic girdle. Churchill Livingstone, Edinburgh

Lewit K 1999 Manipulation in rehabilitation of the motor system, 3rd edn. Butterworths, London

Liebenson C 2000 The trunk extensors and spinal stability. Journal of Bodywork and Movement Therapies 4:246–249

Lin J-P 1994 Physiological maturation of muscles in childhood. Lancet 4:1386–1389

Linton S 2000 Review of psychological risk factors in back and neck pain. Spine 25:1148–1156

Lowe J, Honeyman-Lowe G 1998 Facilitating the decrease in fibromyalgic pain during metabolic rehabilitation. Journal of Bodywork and Movement Therapies 2:208–217

Lum L 1987 Hyperventilation syndromes in medicine and psychiatry. Journal of the Royal Society of Medicine 80:229–231

Luo X, Pietrobon R, Sun S 2004 Estimates and patterns of direct health care expenditures among individuals with back pain in the United States. Spine 29:79–86

McGill S 2004 Functional anatomy of lumbar stability. Proceedings of 5th Interdisciplinary World Congress on Low Back and Pelvic Pain. Melbourne, Australia, p 3–9

Meade T et al 1995 Randomised comparison of chiropractic and hospital outpatient management of low back pain; results from extended follow-up. British Medical Journal 11:349

Moore J, Von Korff M, Cherkin D et al 2000 A randomized trial of a cognitive-behavioral program for enhancing back pain self-care in a primary care setting. Pain 88:45–153

Muller K, Kreutzfeldt A, Schwesig R et al 2003 Hypermobility and chronic back pain. Manuelle Medizin 41:105–109

Nachemson A 1985 Advances in low-back pain. Clinical Orthopaedics and Related Research 200:266–278

Nixon P, Andrews J 1996 A study of anaerobic threshold in chronic fatigue syndrome (CFS). Biological Psychology 43:264

Panjabi M 1992 The stabilizing system of the spine. Part 1. Function, dysfunction, adaptation, and enhancement. Journal of Spinal Disorders 5:383–389

Paris S 1997 Differential diagnosis of lumbar and pelvic pain. In: Vleeming A, Mooney V, Dorman T et al (eds) Movement, stability and low back pain. Churchill Livingstone, Edinburgh

RCGP 1999 Clinical Guidelines for Management of Acute Low Back Pain. Royal College of General Practitioners, London

Selye H 1956 The stress of life. McGraw-Hill, New York

Simons D, Travell J, Simons L 1999 Myofascial pain and dysfunction: the trigger point manual, Vol 1, Upper half of body, 2nd edn. Williams & Wilkins, Baltimore

Snook S, Webster B, McGorry R 1998 The reduction of chronic non-specific low back pain through the control of early morning lumbar flexion. Spine 23:2601–2607

Snook S, Webster B, McGorry R 2002 The reduction of chronic, non-specific low back pain through the control of early morning lumbar flexion: 3-year follow-up. Journal of Occupational Rehabilitation 12:13–20

Travell J, Simons D 1992 Myofascial pain and dysfunction: the trigger point manual, vol 2, the lower extremeties. Williams and Wilkins, Baltimore

Triano J, McGregor M, Hondras M A et al 1995 Manipulative therapy versus education programs in chronic low back pain. Spine 20:948–955

Turk D C, Michenbaum D H, Genest M 1983 Pain and behavioral medicine: a cognitive behavioral perspective. Guildford Press, New York

Van Tulder M, Becker A, Nekkering T et al 2004 European Guidelines for the Management of Acute Non-specific Low Back Pain in Primary Care. Proceedings of the 5th Interdisciplinary World Congress on Low Back and Pelvic Pain, 2004, Melbourne Australia, p 56–79

Vlaeyen J, Crombez G 1999 Fear of movement (re)injury, avoidance and pain disability in chronic low back pain patients. Manual Therapy 4:187–195

Waddell G 1998 The back pain revolution. Churchill Livingstone, Edinburgh

Wall P, Melzack R 1989 Textbook of pain. Churchill Livingstone, Edinburgh

Westhof E, Ernst E 1992 Geschichte der Massage. Deutsche Medizinische Wochenschrift 117:150–153

Wiesinger G, Quittan M et al 1997 Benefit and costs of passive modalities in back pain outpatients: a descriptive study. European Journal of Physical Medicine Rehabilitation 7:182–186

Wilson A 2001 Effective management of musculoskeletal injury. Churchill Livingstone, Edinburgh

Winters J, Crago P (eds) 2000 Biomechanics and neural control of posture and movement. Springer, New York

Woo S Y, Buckwalter J A (eds) 1987 Injury and repair of musculoskeletal soft tissues. American Academy of Orthopedic Surgeons Symposium, Savannah

Chapter 2

Impostor back pain

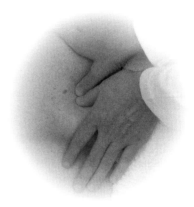

This book is about non-specific back pain – the cause of 97% of all back aches. It is *not* about back pain caused by possibly serious diseases such as cancer, arthritis or deformity. It is also *not* about back pain that obviously derives from disc or facet joint problems or diseases, or about back pain that results from neurological disease.

This does not mean to suggest that massage, and other associated manual methods, cannot offer some relief to people with these more serious causes of back pain, but it strongly suggests that you should be aware of which type of problem you are treating.

As outlined in Chapter 1, non-specific back pain almost always gets better in a matter of weeks or months, and the evidence (also discussed in Chapter 1) is that massage can help in this process. Massage might, in the short term, be able to ease the pain of backache caused by serious conditions, but massage cannot change the course of more serious problems. It is important for the patient's safety, and for your own protection, that if you are in any doubt about the causes of a person's back pain, you should refer the patient for a diagnosis.

In this chapter, we will briefly outline:

1 Imposter symptoms
2 The main pathological causes of back pain
3 Neurological causes of back pain.

The purpose is to clarify those causes that this book does not cover, because our focus is on the vast number of people who suffer unnecessarily from *non-specific* back pain – a condition that research has shown to be commonly helped by appropriate massage and soft tissue treatment (Cherkin et al 2001, Ernst 1999).

GRIEVE'S MASQUERADERS

Grieve (1994) has described conditions which 'masquerade' as others. He says, 'If we take patients off the street, we need ... to be awake to those conditions which may be other than musculoskeletal; this is not 'diagnosis', only an enlightened awareness of when manual or other physical therapy may be ... unsuitable and perhaps foolish. There is also the factor of perhaps delaying more appropriate treatment'. You might become suspicious that a problem is caused by something other than musculoskeletal dysfunction – and seek a definitive diagnosis – when:

- misleading symptoms are reported
- something does not seem quite right regarding the patient's story describing the pain or other symptoms
- your 'gut feeling', instinct, intuition, internal alarm system alerts you. If this happens you should always err on the side of caution and refer onward for another opinion
- the patient reports patterns of activities that aggravate or ease the symptoms that seem unusual and cause you to have doubts about the case being straightforward.

It is important to remember that symptoms can arise from sinister causes (tumors for example) that closely mimic musculoskeletal symptoms, and/or which may coexist alongside actual musculoskeletal dysfunction.

When there is lack of progress in symptoms reduction, or if there are unusual responses to treatment, this should cause you to review the situation.

CAUTIONS: RED AND YELLOW FLAGS

Red flags are signs that may be present, alongside acute back pain, that suggest that other factors than musculoskeletal dysfunction are operating. In most people, there are no obvious pathological features associated with their back pain, but:

- around 4% have compression fractures (probably with osteoporosis as a background to that)
- 1% have tumors as the cause of the problem
- between 1 and 3% of people with acute back pain have prolapsed discs (Deyo et al 1992).

Multiple causes of identical pain

Giles (2003) has demonstrated how a number of very different conditions can produce back pain in precisely the same place (Fig. 2.1).

Pain in the area shown in Figure 2.1 can be the result of:

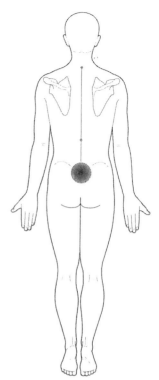

Figure 2.1 Localized presenting complaint site. (From Giles 2003.)

- Carcinoma of the pancreas (see Fig. 2.3)
- Inflammatory arthropathy
- Abdominal aneurysm
- Leg length inequality.

Pain distribution as shown in Figure 2.2 can be the result of:

- Intervertebral disc protrusion (see Fig. 2.4)
- Sacroiliac joint dysfunction
- A small aortic aneurysm
- Pain following discectomy
- Spondylolisthesis (see Fig. 2.5)
- Cauda equina syndrome
- Tethered cord syndrome
- Lumbar neuroma
- Perineural fibrosis.

'Red flags' for impostor (masquerader) symptoms

The red and yellow flag lists, given below, are derived from the document *European Guidelines for the Management of Acute Non-specific Low Back Pain in Primary Care* (RCGP 1999). Red flags suggest (but do not prove) the possibility of more serious pathology.

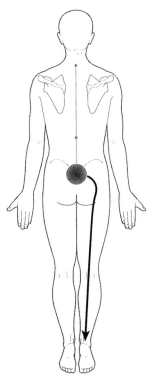

Figure 2.2   Presenting complaint, radiating pain pattern. (From Giles 2003.)

Suspicion or recognition of red flags emerges from the person's history and symptoms.

If any of the signs listed below are present, further investigation should be suggested before treatment starts, particularly to exclude infection, inflammatory disease or cancer (RCGP 1999).

- The acute back pain started when the person was <20 years or >55 years old
- There is an associated recent history of violent trauma such as a motor vehicle accident or a fall
- There seems to be a constant progressive, non-mechanical pain that is characterized by no relief being experienced with bed-rest
- There is thoracic pain accompanying the back pain
- The patient reports a past history of malignancy
- There is a history of prolonged use of corticosteroids (such as cortisone)
- The patient has a history of drug abuse, taking of immunosuppressive medication, or a diagnosis of being HIV positive
- The back pain is accompanied by systemic 'unwellness', and/or unexplained weight loss

- There are widespread neurological symptoms. For example, there may have been changes in bladder control, or widespread or progressive limb weakness, or changes in gait
- There is obvious structural deformity such as scoliosis
- The back pain is accompanied by fever.

Note: It is probable that one form of massage or another would be useful for back pain relating to all or any of these signs and symptoms, but this should not be offered until the real nature of the problem has been investigated. It would be both unethical and unprofessional to delay such investigation.

'Yellow flags'

Unlike the possibly pathological signs that the red flags represent, yellow flags suggest psychosocial factors that 'increase the risk of developing, or perpetuating chronic pain and long-term disability' (Van Tulder et al 2004).

Examples include (Kendall et al 1997):

- Inappropriate attitudes about back pain, such as the belief that back pain is actually harmful and potentially disabling; or that bed-rest is all that is needed rather than performing specific beneficial exercises. One of the first and most important lessons people need to learn is that '*hurt does not necessarily mean harm*'
- Inappropriate pain-behavior, for example reducing activity levels or 'fear-avoidance'
- Compensation (the possibility of financial gain if back pain continues), and/or work-related issues (for example poor work satisfaction and the 'benefit' of time away from it)
- Background emotional problems such as depression, anxiety, high stress levels.

SPECIFIC DISEASES OR CONDITIONS THAT INVOLVE, OR MIMIC, BACK PAIN

- A degenerative (e.g. arthritic) hip can refer pain beyond the hip area, resulting in pain in the groin, sacroiliac joint (SIJ) and lower back
- Trochanteric bursitis usually causes hip pain
- Lumbar zygapophysial (facet) syndrome can refer pain to the buttock and SIJ, as well as the pain wrapping around the hip to the anterior thigh
- Ovarian cysts, fibroid tumors, and endometriosis can sometimes refer pain to the hip or SIJ area
- Inflammation or dysfunction of the fallopian tubes may cause SIJ pain because the suspensory ligament of the fallopian tube attaches to the front of the SIJ.

Other 'impostor' symptoms that replicate or produce low back pain

Mense and Simons (2001) describe general regions of the back that may become painful in response to organ diseases:

- *Acute kidney pain*: The flank area, running from the lower ribs down towards the pelvic crest and round to the anterior superior iliac spine may all develop a severe deep ache that does not change with movement or when posture is modified. Abdominal trigger point activity can be an additional source
- *Pain which closely resembles acute thoracolumbar dysfunction* can be the result of stones in the ureter ('renal colic')
- *Acute pancreatitis*: Along with acute abdominal 'stabbing' pain, there is a radiating pain in the lower thoracic spine spreading downwards. Spasm may also occur in the lower chest wall
- Almost any abdominal disorder (such as peptic ulcer, colon cancer, abdominal arterial disease) can produce pain in the back. Therefore, all other reported symptoms, especially those involving the digestive system, should be evaluated alongside the musculoskeletal assessment. Viscerosomatic pain should be considered, especially if back pain and symptoms associated with internal organs coincide (Fig. 2.3)
- A hiatal hernia (involving the diaphragm) is usually associated with bilateral thoracic and shoulder pain
- Waddell (1998) suggests that cauda equina syndrome (involving a cluster of fine nerves at the end of the spinal cord) and/or widespread neurological disorders, should be considered if the patient with low back pain reports difficulty with urination (desire for, or frequent urination, or inability to urinate at times), and/or fecal incontinence. A *saddle formation* area of anesthesia may be reported around the anus, perineum or genitals. There may be accompanying motor weakness in the legs, together with gait disturbance. Immediate specialist referral is called for with any such symptoms
- You should be suspicious of ankylosing spondylitis, or other chronic inflammatory conditions, if the symptoms of low backache arrive (usually in a male) slowly but progressively, before 40 years of age, especially if there is a family history; extreme stiffness in the morning; constant stiffness involving all movements of the spine and peripheral joint pain and restriction. There may also be associated colitis, iritis and/or skin problems such as psoriasis
- The patient with angina pain usually presents with chest, anterior cervical and (usually left) arm pain.

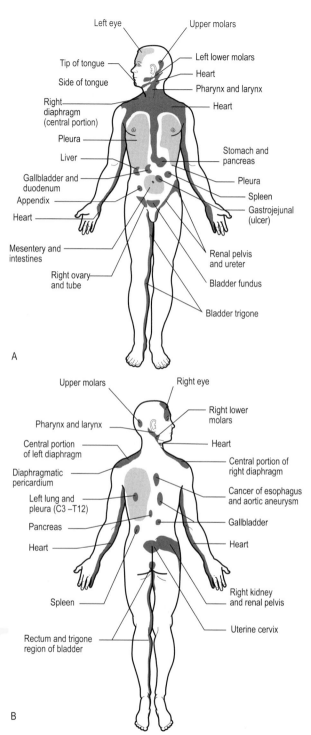

Figure 2.3 Pain referred from viscera. (A) Anterior view. (B) Posterior view. (Adapted from Rothstein et al 1991.) (From Chaitow and DeLany 2000.)

Thoracic facet or disc conditions can mimic angina, as can active trigger point activity. Those factors that are reported as aggravating or easing the symptoms can usually offer clues as to whether the condition is cardiac related, or whether the symptoms are caused by biomechanical influences

- A dysfunctional or diseased gall bladder commonly refers pain to the mid-thoracic area uni- or bilaterally, or to the shoulder and tip of the scapula on the same side
- Sacroiliac and right buttock pain may be produced by perforation of the ilium in regional ileitis (Crohn's disease)
- Severe low back pain (possibly referring to the testicles) may be associated with an aneurysm that is about to rupture
- If a patient has a background of coronary, pulmonary or bronchial disease, the vertebral veins may have become varicosed, leading to an ill-defined backache
- Osteitis deformans (Paget's disease) may present with a constant aching pain but may be symptomless. Needle biopsy is necessary for confirmation of a diagnosis
- The filament at the end of the dural tube, the filum terminale, may be involved in a tethering lesion, especially in adolescents during the 'growth spurt' years, with symptoms of back pain.

Where else might pain derive from in low back pain problems?

- Fatigued and ischemic musculature (and tendons) – established by tests which evaluate unbalanced firing patterns, such as prone hip extension test and side-lying hip abduction test. See Chapter 4 for these functional assessments
- Muscle shortness, which is usually obviously related to postural imbalances such as the lower crossed syndrome (see Fig. 4.9) and further established by specific muscle shortness evaluations
- Fibrosis and other soft tissue changes (established during massage, neuromuscular technique (NMT) and other palpation procedures). Treatment protocols will depend on the nature of the dysfunctional pattern, and might include deep connective tissue work, stretching methods such as muscle energy technique (MET) and myofascial release (MFR), as well as rehabilitation exercises (see Chs 7 and 8)
- Myofascial trigger points – established by NMT and other palpation methods and treated by appropriate deactivation strategies including NMT, integrated neuromuscular inhibition technique (INIT), MET, positional release technique (PRT), acupuncture, etc. (see Ch. 7)

- Instability involving spinal ligament weakness – established by history and/or assessment. Ligamentous weakness is a common cause of instability (Paris 1997). Ligamentous weakness pain usually starts as a dull ache, spreading slowly throughout the day to muscles that are taking over the ligament's role as stabilizers. People who habitually self-manipulate ('cracking themselves') may obtain short-term relief, but actually increase the degree of instability. Treatment should include reestablishing optimal muscular balance, core stability exercises (see Ch. 8)
- Degenerative discs may cause motor weakness and loss of sensation. These may be diagnosed by use of scan evidence (Fig. 2.4). Treatment depends on the degree of acuteness/chronicity. Traction might be used but this is not universally approved (Paris 1997). Bed-rest may be essential in some cases, if acute swelling of soft tissues in the area of disc protrusion has occurred. In the sub-acute stage postural reeducation, mild stretching, core stability and other specific exercises (such as extension

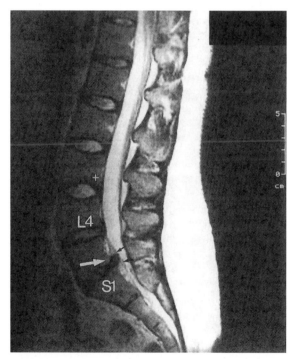

Figure 2.4   An MRI T2-weighted sagittal lumbar spine scan showing the moderately large central disc protrusion at the L5–S1 level (white arrow) that may be confined by the posterior longitudinal ligament which is displaced posteriorly. The moderately severe degree of compression on the anterior aspect of the dural tube/thecal sac is clearly visible (black arrows). Note that the L5–S1 intervertebral disc shows more advanced desiccation than does the L4–5 disc. (From Giles 2003.)

exercises to re-establish lordosis if this has been lost) may be prescribed. Surgery should only be considered if neurological signs are evident

- Involvement of zygapophyseal facet joints as a cause of back pain requires careful assessment. Facet dysfunction might include facet capsule synovitis, facet capsule entrapment, facet blockage due to meniscus or loose body entrapment, or degenerative arthrosis of the facet joint. Treatment of facet joint problems may include rest and/or manipulation or pain killing injections
- SIJ capsules and ligaments – the sacroiliac joint and its ligaments are a common source of low back pain (see Ch. 5)
- Congenital anomalies such as spondylolisthesis (where a vertebral segment has 'slipped' forward on the one below) can be established by X-ray or scan. Unless there are neurological signs, spondylolisthesis is best treated by encouraging improved posture, rebalancing of the low back/pelvic musculature, and core stabilization protocols (see Ch. 8). If neurological signs accompany a spondylolisthesis, surgery and possibly fusion may be required (Fig. 2.5)
- Stenosis (narrowing) of the spinal canal or lateral foramen is evaluated by means of signs and symptoms and scan evidence. Stenosis may produce neurological symptoms aggravated by exercise and relieved by forward bending
- Arthritic changes. Signs and symptoms and history, as well as X-ray or scan evidence, confirms the presence of arthritic changes, including conditions such as lupus, ankylosing spondylitis, rheumatoid and osteoarthritis. Manual therapy may offer pain relief and circulatory and drainage enhancement
- Low back pain may be a feature of widespread conditions in which pain is a primary feature, such as fibromyalgia, where bodywork plays a role in palliative care.

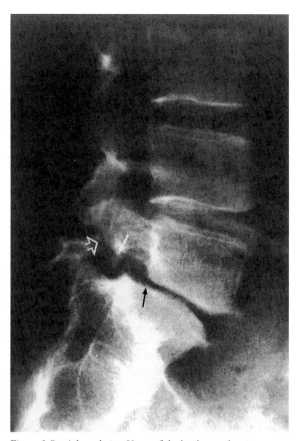

Figure 2.5   A lateral view X-ray of the lumbosacral region showing grade 1 spondylolisthesis of L5 on S1 with advanced thinning of the intervertebral disc at this level and osteophytic lipping at the anterior margins of the L5 and S1 bodies. The open arrow shows the fractured pars interarticularis. The white arrow indicates the bone spicule projecting into the right L5–S1 intervertebral foramen. The black arrow shows the degree of spondylolisthesis, i.e. the L5 body as moved approximately one-quarter of the distance along the sacral body, hence the grade 1 classification according to Myerding's (1932) classification. (Giles & Singer 1997, Yochum & Rowe 1996.) (From Giles 2003.)

LEWIT'S ADVICE

Karel Lewit (1992) suggests that, apart from their local significance in terms of pain, and their influence on target areas, trigger points can have a clinical significance due to their links with certain pathologies, for example triggers in:

- the thigh adductors may indicate hip pathology
- iliacus may indicate lesions/subluxation of segments L5–S1 (coccyx)
- piriformis may indicate lesions/subluxation of segment L4–5 (coccyx)
- rectus femoris may indicate lesions/subluxation of L3–4 (hip)
- psoas may indicate lesions/subluxation of the thoraco-lumbar junction (T10–L1)
- erector spinae muscles may indicate lesions/subluxation of a corresponding spinal level
- rectus abdominis may indicate problems at the xiphoid, pubis or low back.

NERVE ROOT PAIN

This commonly produces sciatic type pain and causes can include disc prolapse, stenosis of the spine, scar formation, or more complex neurological disorders. As a rule, nerve root pain involves pain along the sciatic distribution, down the leg and including the foot, which is more intense than the accompanying back pain. There is commonly a degree of numbness in the same areas as the pain. If neurological symptoms or signs affect several nerve roots or both legs, then there may be a more widespread neurological disorder. This may present as unsteadiness or gait disturbance.

One of the clearest signs of neural involvement in low back/sciatic pain is the straight leg raising test (see Ch. 4), which aggravates and/or reproduces the painful symptoms (Butler & Gifford 1989).

DISTORTIONS AND ANOMALIES

If abnormal structural features are noted on standing examination, such as scoliosis or marked kyphosis, it is important to observe whether this remains evident during prone positioning.

- If it does not remain in prone positioning, i.e. the spinal distortion reduces or normalizes when the patient lies face down, then it represents muscular contraction/spasm. A true scoliosis will remain evident even under anesthetic

- If it does remain in prone positioning, the cause may be structural, or may be muscular, since a long term, fixated, muscularly induced scoliosis may also remain in non-weight bearing position.

KEY POINTS

- While massage and associated soft tissue methods may offer short-term pain relief for almost all forms of back pain, it is only useful in relation to speeding recovery in non-specific back pain
- If there are red or yellow flag suspicions, it is important to have the patient seek a firm diagnosis rather than possibly offering short-term pain relief for a problem that needs urgent attention elsewhere
- There are a variety of congenital, structural, neurological, pathological and degenerative causes for the small proportion of back pain that has specific causes
- Identical localized low back pain, with or without referral into the lower limb, can derive from a variety of different conditions, making differential diagnosis essential for the safety of both the patient and the therapist.

References

Butler D, Gifford L 1989 Adverse mechanical tensions in the nervous system. Physiotherapy 75:622–629

Chaitow L, DeLany J 2000 Clinical applications of neuromuscular technique, Volume 1. Churchill Livingstone, Edinburgh

Cherkin D, Eisenberg D, Sherman K et al 2001 Randomized trial comparing traditional Chinese medical acupuncture, therapeutic massage, and self-care education for chronic low back pain. Archives of Internal Medicine 161:1081–1088

Deyo R, Rainville J, Kent D 1992 What can the history and physical examination tell us about low back pain? Journal of the American Medical Association 268:760–765

Ernst E 1999 Massage therapy for low back pain: a systematic review. Journal of Pain and Symptom Management 17(1):65–69

Giles L 2003 50 Challenging spinal pain syndrome cases. Butterworth-Heinemann, Edinburgh

Giles L G F 1997 Miscellaneous pathological and developmental (anomalous) conditions. In: Giles L G F, Singer KP (eds) Clinical anatomy and management of low back pain, Vol 1. Butterworth-Heinemann, Oxford, pp 196–216

Grieve G 1994 The masqueraders. In: Boyling J D, Palastanga N (eds) Grieve's modern manual therapy of the vertebral column, 2nd edn. Churchill Livingstone, Edinburgh

Kendall N, Linton S, Main C 1997 Guide to assessing psychosocial yellow flags in acute low back pain. Accident Rehabilitation & Compensation Insurance Corporation of New Zealand, Wellington

Lewit K 1992 Manipulative therapy in rehabilitation of the locomotor system, 2nd edn. Butterworths, London

Mense S, Simons D 2001 Muscle pain. Lippincott Williams & Wilkins, Baltimore, p 142–143

Paris S 1997 Differential diagnosis of lumbar and pelvic pain. In: Vleeming A, Mooney V, Dorman T et al (eds) Movement, stability and low back pain. Churchill Livingstone, New York

RCGP 1999 European Guidelines for the Management of Acute Non-specific Low Back Pain in Primary Care. Royal College of General Practitioners, London.

Rothstein J et al 1991 Rehabilitation specialists' handbook. FA Davis, Philadelphia

Van Tulder M, Becker A, Nekkering T et al 2004 European Guidelines for the Management of Acute Nonspecific Low Back Pain in Primary Care. Proceedings of the 5th Interdisciplinary World Congress on Low Back and Pelvic Pain. Melbourne, Australia, p 56–79

Waddell G 1998 The back pain revolution. Churchill Livingstone, Edinburgh

Yochum T R, Rowe L J 1996 Essentials of skeletal radiology, 2nd edn. Williams and Wilkins, Baltimore, pp 237–372

Chapter 3

How much pain is there, where is it and where might it be coming from?

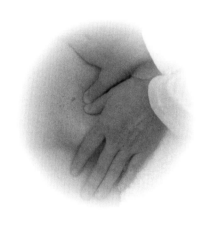

TRIGGER POINTS

Pain in the back can frequently be the result of referred pain from active myofascial trigger points (TrPs), and the maps in Figure 3.1A–I can help to identify where these might be located.

Working backwards from the site of the pain, it is a simple matter to identify the probable location of the trigger point(s) that may be feeding pain into the distressed tissues (Simons et al 1999).

Definitions of active and latent trigger points are found in Box 3.1.

TRIGGER POINT PALPATION SITES

Raymond Nimmo (1957), a pioneer of the early years of research into trigger points compiled useful information as to where to palpate for trigger points referring to specific areas:

- 'Firm pressure on the superior border of the sacrum, between the iliac spine and the sacral spinous process, produces pressure on the SI ligament. Move the contact superiorly and inferiorly searching for sensitivity' (Nimmo 1966).

Triggers here are involved in all low back syndromes and 50% of all patients, according to Nimmo.

As in all descriptions given (below), it is suggested that you search both sides.

- Press just superiorly to the sacral base adjacent to the spine, medial to PSIS. This is the iliolumbar ligament. Heavy pressure is required to find triggers which are involved in most low back problems.

Search both sides. A 90% incidence is reported.

- Hook your thumb under the sacrosciatic and sacrotuberous ligaments medial and inferior to the ischial tuberosity, lifting and stretching laterally if painful.

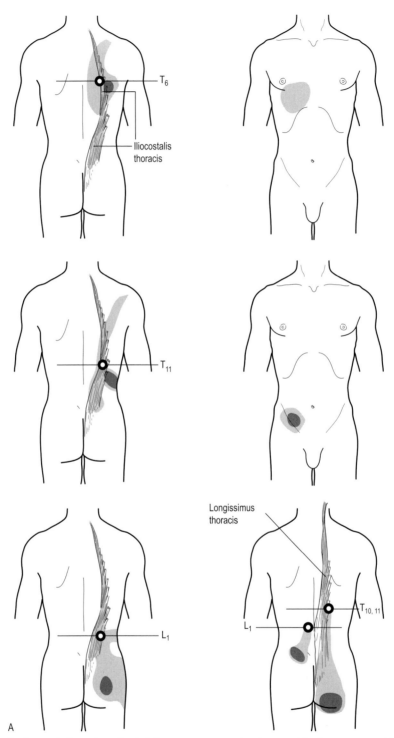

Figure 3.1 (A) Superficial paraspinal muscles collectively known as erector spinae have combined target zones which refer across most of the posterior surface of the body and anteriorly as well. (From Chaitow and DeLany 2000.)

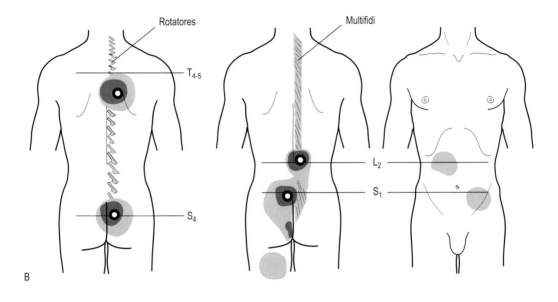

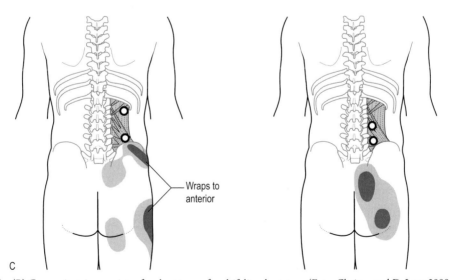

Figure 3.1, cont'd   (B) Composite trigger point referral patterns of multifidi and rotators. (From Chaitow and DeLany 2000.)
(C) Quadratus lumborum trigger points refer into SI joint, lower buttocks and wrap laterally along the iliac crest and hip region. A referral pattern into the lower abdomen region is not illustrated. (Adapted from Travell and Simons (1992), Fig. 4.1A, B.) (From Chaitow and DeLany 2002.)

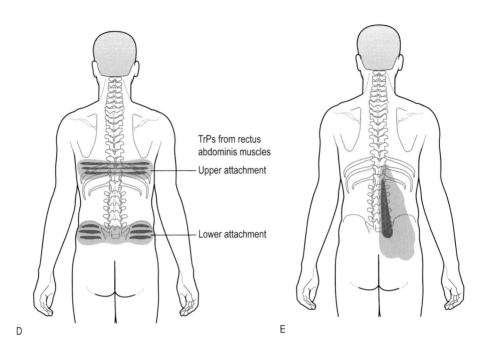

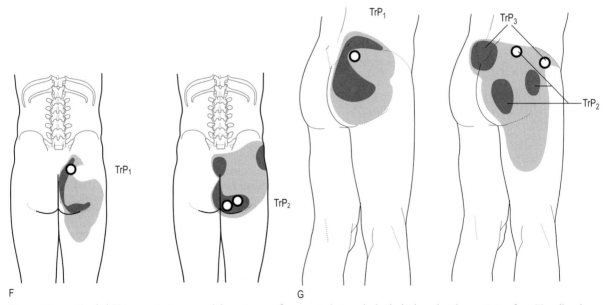

Figure 3.1, cont'd   (D) Trigger point in rectus abdominis can refer posteriorly into the back. (Adapted with permission from Travell and Simons (1992).) (From Chaitow and DeLany 2002.) (E) Referral pattern for iliopsoas may continue further than illustrated into the sacrum and proximal medial buttocks. Additionally, it may refer into the upper anterior thigh (not illustrated). (Adapted with permission from Travell and Simons (1992).) (From Chaitow and DeLany 2002.) (F) The referred patterns of the gluteus maximus include the sacroiliac joint, sacrum, hip, ischium and coccyx. They can be the source of low backache, lumbago and coccygodynia. (Adapted with permission from Travell and Simons (1992).) (From Chaitow and DeLany 2002.) (G) Target referral zones for gluteus medius trigger points. (Adapted with permission from Travell and Simons (1992).) (From Chaitow and DeLany 2002.)

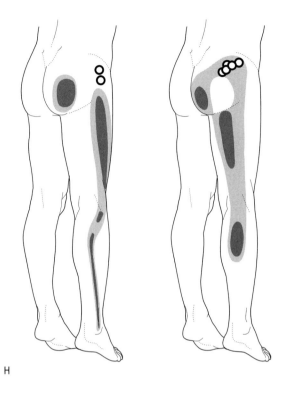

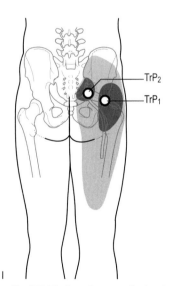

Figure 3.1, cont'd (H) The 'pseudo-sciatica' referral patterns for gluteus minimus trigger points (From Chaitow and DeLany 2002.) (I) Awareness of the course of the sciatic nerve should be ever present on the practitioner's mind as examination of this region takes place. Target zone of referral of piriformis is also shown. (Adapted with permission from Travell & Simons 1992.) (From Chaitow and DeLany 2002.)

Nimmo reports a 30% incidence of triggers in these sites.

Note: Nimmo used a palm-held, rubber-tipped wooden T-bar, in order to apply pressure to areas requiring high poundage, such as the iliolumbar ligament.

- Medial pressure is applied by the thumb to the lateral border of quadratus lumborum, avoiding pressure on the tips of transverse processes, starting below the last rib down to the pelvic rim. A 'gummy' feel will be noted if contracture exists (plus sensitivity) in contrast to the resilient, homogeneous feel of normal muscle. Triggers here are often associated with low back problems. If latissimus dorsi is also involved, pain may radiate to the shoulder or arm.

An 80% incidence of trigger point activity is reported in these muscles, according to Nimmo's research.

- Search the area below the posterior aspect of the ilia for noxious points associated with gluteal muscles generally
- Search the central region of the belly of gluteus medius for triggers which can produce sciatic-type pain.

A 90% incidence is reported.

- Search midway between the trochanters and the superior crest of the ilium, in the central portion of gluteus minimus where a trigger point affecting the lateral aspect of, e.g. the foot, or duplicating sciatic-type pain, is common.

This also has a 90% incidence of triggers, as opposed to gluteus maximus, which produces active triggers in only 4% of patients with back pain.

- The point of intersection, where imaginary lines drawn from the posterior superior iliac spine (PSIS) to the trochanter, and from the ischial tuberosity to the anterior superior iliac spine (ASIS) meet, is the access point for contact with the insertion of the piriformis muscle
- If the line from the ASIS is taken to the coccyx, the intersection is over the belly of the piriformis. These two points should be palpated; if sensitivity is noted, the muscle requires treatment. Sciatic-type pain distribution to the knee is a common referred symptom.

A 40% incidence of triggers is reported by Nimmo.

- Hamstring trigger points lie about a hand's width above the knee joint in about 20% of patients
- With the supine patient's knees flexed, the therapist stands on the side to be examined. Place finger pads

---

Box 3.1   Active and latent trigger points

The pain characteristics of an active myofascial trigger point are:

- When pressure is applied, active trigger points are painful and either refer (i.e. symptoms are felt at a distance from the point of pressure) or radiate (i.e. symptoms spread from the point of pressure)
- Symptoms that are referred or that radiate include pain, tingling, numbness, burning, itching or other sensations, and most importantly, in an active trigger these symptoms are recognizable (familiar) to the person.

There are other signs of an active trigger point ('jump sign', palpable indications such as a taut band, fasciculation etc.).

The pain characteristics of a latent myofascial trigger point are:

- Commonly, the individual is not aware of the existence of a latent point until it is pressed (that is, unlike an active point, a latent one seldom produces spontaneous pain)
- When pressure is applied to a latent point it is usually painful, and it may refer (i.e. symptoms are felt at a distance from the point of pressure), or radiate (i.e. symptoms spread from the point of pressure)
- If the symptoms, whether pain, tingling, numbness, burning, itching or other sensations, are not familiar, or perhaps are sensations that the person used to have in the past, but has not experienced recently, then this is a latent myofascial trigger point.

Progression
Latent trigger points may become active trigger points at any time, perhaps becoming a 'common, everyday headache' or adding to, or expanding, the pattern of pain already being experienced for other reasons.

The change from latent to active may occur when the tissues are overused, strained by overload, chilled, stretched (particularly if this is rapid), shortened, traumatized (as in a motor vehicle accident or a fall or blow) or when other perpetuating factors (such as poor nutrition or shallow breathing) provide less than optimal conditions of tissue health.

Active trigger points may become latent trigger points with their referral patterns subsiding for brief or prolonged periods of time. They may then be reactivated with their referral patterns returning for no apparent reason.

Embryonic points
Any sensitive point in the soft tissues, that hurts unusually on pressure, but which does not radiate or refer, is termed an embryonic trigger point.

This is a disturbed or dysfunctional region of soft tissue that, over time, with sufficient additional stress input (overuse etc.), may become first a latent, and eventually, an active trigger point.

Attachment and central points
When a trigger point is situated near the center (belly) of a muscle, near the motor end-point, it is known as a central point. When it is situated close to the insertion/attachment of a muscle, it is known as an attachment point.

---

just superior to the ASIS, pressing towards the floor and then towards the feet, allowing access under the pelvic crest to contact the iliacus muscle. A gliding contact, followed by flexing of the contact fingers allows searching of this area for triggers.

A 90% incidence of triggers is reported by Nimmo.

- Access to the psoas muscle is suggested from the lateral margin of rectus abdominis, allowing finger contact to pass under the sigmoid on the left, and under the caecum on the right. This accesses the belly of psoas in non-obese patients. Another access is directly towards the spine from the midline (patient with flexed knees), some 7.5 cm below the umbilicus. On approaching the spine (denser feel), finger pad contact slides laterally over the body of the lumbar vertebrae (2, 3 or 4) towards the opposite side. This will contact the origin of psoas, a common site for triggers.

A 50–70% incidence of triggers is reported by Nimmo.

- Abductor longus and pectineus can be contacted with the patient in the same position, as thumbs glide along the abductor towards pubic attachment and then laterally to contact pectineus.

An incidence of 50% of patients have triggers in this muscle.

- Tensor fascia lata is best contacted with the patient side-lying, affected leg straight, supported by the flexed other leg. Triggers here can produce sciatic-type pain.

A 70% incidence of triggers is reported by Nimmo.

VISCERA AND BACK PAIN

We have seen in the previous chapter that impostor pain exists, sometimes arising in visceral organs and referring to the back. Refer back to Figure 2.3 for a sense of just how important it is for the patient (and for you) for an accurate diagnosis to be made. You should never feel embarrassed to say to the patient that you want to be certain of the cause before starting treatment, and then to refer the patient to someone licensed to make that diagnosis. Your professionalism will be respected, and once you have the diagnosis, you will have the confidence to commence treatment with a reassured patient.

PELVIC PAIN

Pelvic pain, and problems of urgency and incontinence, may also at times be related to trigger points, although of course there may be many other causes of these symptoms, including infection, gynecological disease, pregnancy, weight problems, etc. Since the early 1950s there have been reports that symptoms such as cystitis could be created by trigger points in the abdominal muscles (Kelsey 1951). Travell & Simons (1983), the leading researchers into trigger points, reported that:

> Urinary frequency, urinary urgency and 'kidney' pain may be referred from trigger points in the skin of the lower abdominal muscles. Injection of an old appendectomy scar ... has relieved frequency and urgency, and increased the bladder capacity significantly.

More recent research confirms this, and has shown that symptoms such as cystitis can often be relieved manually, as well as by injection (Oyama et al 2004, Weiss 2001).

MEASURING THE PAIN

Wolfe et al (1995) showed that although approximately 60% of women can tolerate 4 kg (±8 lbs) of pressure before reporting pain, approximately 90% of men can tolerate this amount of pressure without feeling what they would describe as pain. Less than 5% of women can tolerate 12 kg (±25 lbs) of pressure, while nearly 50% of men can do so. This gender difference is well worth remembering when using pressure to test pain levels.

It is important to have ways of easily recording the person's present sense of pain (Melzack & Katz 1999), so that there is a record that can be compared with treatment progress.

You need to know:

- where the pain is
- what it feels like to the patient (words such as ache, sharp, burning, etc.)
- what other symptoms (inflammation for example, or a fever) accompany the pain

- whether any of the symptoms are constant or fluctuating
- what aggravates the pain and what makes it easier
- the times of day when pain is most obvious (In bed at night? When moving about? After moving about and sitting?)
- what activities are prevented by the pain ('I cannot (or it is difficult to) walk, sit down, carry anything', etc.).

Tools for measuring pain

There are a variety of 'tools' that can help to record symptoms such as pain, ranging from questionnaires, to simple paper based measuring scales, as well as instruments such as a pressure gauge, an algometer.

There are various types of algometer. Some are simple spring-loaded, hand-held devices, while others use digital technology. Algometers are discussed further below.

Rating scales (Fig. 3.2A–C)
The simplest measuring device, the verbal rating scale (VRS) (Fig. 3.2A), records on paper, or a computer, what a patient reports, i.e. whether there is 'no pain', 'mild pain', 'moderate pain', 'severe pain' or 'agonizing pain' (Jensen & Karoly 1991).

A numerical rating scale (NRS)   This method uses a series of numbers (0–100, or 0–10)

- No pain would equal 0
- Worst pain possible would equal the highest number on the scale.

The patient is asked to apply a numerical value to the pain. This is recorded along with the date.

Using an NRS (Fig. 3.2B), is a common and fairly accurate method for measuring the intensity of pain, but does not take account of the 'meaning' the patient gives to the pain (Hong et al 1996).

The visual analogue scale (VAS)   This widely used method consists of a 10 cm line drawn on paper, with marks at each end, and at each cm.

- The 0 end of the line equals no pain at all
- The 10 cm end equals the worst pain possible.

The patient marks the line at the level of their pain. The VAS (Fig. 3.2C), can be used to measure progress by comparing the pain scores over time. The VAS has been found to be accurate when used for anyone over the age of 5 years.

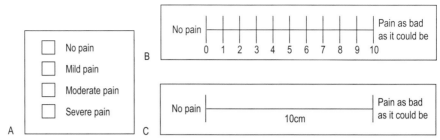

Figure 3.2 (A) A verbal rating scale. The patient is instructed to mark the verbal description that best represents their pain. (B) A numerical rating scale. The patient is instructed to mark the numbered vertical line as appropriate. (C) A horizontal visual analogue scale for pain intensity. (After Kolt and Andersen 2004.)

Questionnaires

A variety of questionnaires exist, such as the McGill Pain Questionnaire (Fig. 3.3), the Short McGill Questionnaire, and many others. The shorter version lists a number of words that describe pain (such as throbbing, shooting, stabbing, heavy, sickening, fearful). The use of such questionnaires requires training so that accurate interpretation can be made of the patient's answers, therefore, apart from acknowledging that they can be very useful, the McGill (and other) question-naires will not be discussed in this book. There are a number of ways of getting further information, the simplest being to conduct a web-search using the 'McGill questionnaire' for the keywords.

Pain drawings

It can be useful for the patient to color the areas of their pain on a simple outline of the human body, using a red pencil (Fig. 3.4A).

The patient should write single word descriptions of the pain in different areas: throbbing, aching, etc., or a simple code can be used, for example:

- xx = burning pain
- !! = stabbing pain
- 00 = aching, and so on.

This records both the location, and the nature, of the person's pain, and can be compared with similar records at future visits.

The shaded or colored areas can be very useful when searching for trigger points, in combination with the body maps provided earlier in this chapter.

A single sheet of paper can easily contain a VAS, a shortened McGill Questionnaire, as well as a series of simple questions such as those illustrated in Figure 3.4B.

Pain threshold

Applying pressure safely requires sensitivity. We need to be able to sense when tissue tension/resistance is being 'met', as we palpate, and when tension is being overcome.

When applying pressure you may ask the patient: 'Does it hurt?', 'Does it refer?' To make sense of the answer it is important to have an idea of how much pressure you are using.

The term 'pain threshold' is used to describe the least amount of pressure needed to produce a report of pain, and/or referred symptoms, when a trigger point is being compressed (Fryer & Hodgson 2005).

It is important to know how much pressure is required to produce pain, and/or referred symptoms, and whether the amount of pressure being used has changed after treatment, or whether the pain threshold is different the next time the patient comes for treatment.

It would not be helpful to hear: 'Yes it still hurts' only because you are pressing much harder!

When testing for trigger point activity, we should be able to apply a moderate amount of force, just enough to cause no more than a sense of pressure (not pain) in normal tissues, and to be always able to apply the same amount of effort whenever we test in this way. We should be able to apply enough pressure to produce the trigger point referral pain, and know that the same pressure, after treatment, no longer causes pain referral.

How can a person learn to apply a particular amount of pressure, and no more?
It has been shown that, using a simple technology (such as bathroom scales), physical therapy students can be taught to accurately produce specific degrees of pressure on request. Students are tested applying

McGill Pain Questionnaire

Patient's name _____ Date _____ Time _____ am/pm

PRI: S _____ A _____ E _____ M _____ PRI(T) _____ PPI _____
(1–10)   (11–15)   (16)   (17–20)   (1–20)

1 FLICKERING	11 TIRING
QUIVERING	EXHAUSTING
PULSING	12 SICKENING
THROBBING	SUFFOCATING
BEATING	13 FEARFUL
POUNDING	FRIGHTFUL
2 JUMPING	TERRIFYING
FLASHING	14 PUNISHING
SHOOTING	GRUELLING
3 PRICKING	CRUEL
BORING	VICIOUS
DRILLING	KILLING
STABBING	15 WRETCHED
LANCINATING	BLINDING
4 SHARP	16 ANNOYING
CUTTING	TROUBLESOME
LACERATING	MISERABLE
5 PINCHING	INTENSE
PRESSING	UNBEARABLE
GNAWING	17 SPREADING
CRAMPING	RADIATING
CRUSHING	PENETRATING
6 TUGGING	PIERCING
PULLING	18 TIGHT
WRENCHING	NUMB
7 HOT	DRAWING
BURNING	SQUEEZING
SCALDING	TEARING
SEARING	19 COOL
8 TINGLING	COLD
ITCHY	FREEZING
SMARTING	20 NAGGING
STINGING	NAUSEATING
9 DULL	AGONIZING
SORE	DREADFUL
HURTING	TORTURING
ACHING	**PPI**
HEAVY	0 NO PAIN
10 TENDER	1 MILD
TAUT	2 DISCOMFORTING
RASPING	3 DISTRESSING
SPLITTING	4 HORRIBLE
	5 EXCRUCIATING

BRIEF · MOMENTARY · TRANSIENT
RHYTHMIC · PERIODIC · INTERMITTENT
CONTINUOUS · STEADY · CONSTANT

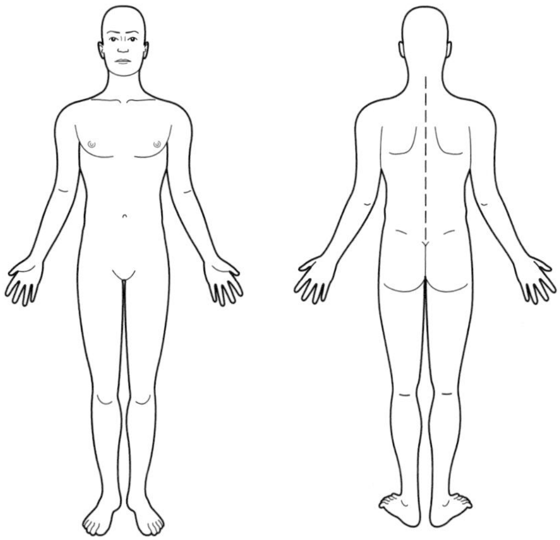

E = EXTERNAL

I = INTERNAL

COMMENTS:

Figure 3.3 McGill Pain Questionnaire. The rank values for each descriptor fall into four main groups: S, sensory; A, affective; E, evaluative; M, miscellaneous. PRI, pain rating index, is the sum of the rank values; PPI, present pain index, is based on a scale of 0–5 (from Melzack R 1975 Pain, 1, The McGill Pain Questionnaire: Major properties and scoring methods, p 227–299, with permission from the International Society for the Study of Pain).

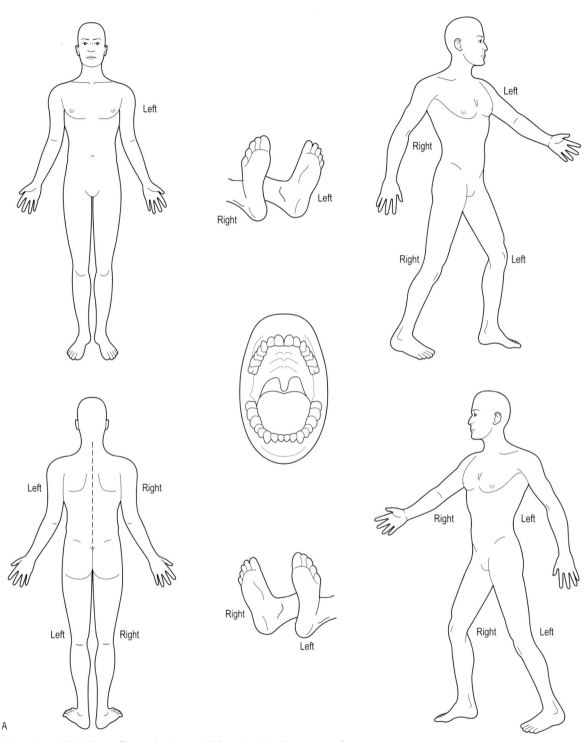

Figure 3.4   (A) Outlines of human body onto which patient sketches patterns of pain.

NAME _____   DATE _____

Please tick any of the words that describe your pain under the column that describes its intensity.

	None	Mild	Moderate	Severe
Throbbing				
Shooting				
Stabbing				
Cramping				
Gnawing				
Hot-Burning				
Aching				
Heavy				
Tender				
Splitting				
Tiring-Exhausting				
Sickening				
Fearful				
Punishing-Cruel				

Your Pain is:

On Most Days ..... No Pain / Mild / Discomforting / Distressing / Horrible / Excruciating

At Its Worst .... No Pain / Mild / Discomforting / Distressing / Horrible / Excruciating

At Its Best .... No Pain / Mild / Discomforting / Distressing / Horrible / Excruciating

TODAY No Pain / Mild / Discomforting / Distressing / Horrible / Excruciating

How many hours of the day are you in pain? ....

How many days per week are you in pain? ....

How many weeks per year are you in pain? ....

What Drugs Have You Taken Today? ....

....

Your Pain Today - Tick along scale below

No Pain [_____ **] Worst Possible Pain**

PLEASE DRAW YOUR PAIN

xxx	Burning	= =	Numbness
!!	Stabbing	**	Cramping
oo	Aching	?	Other

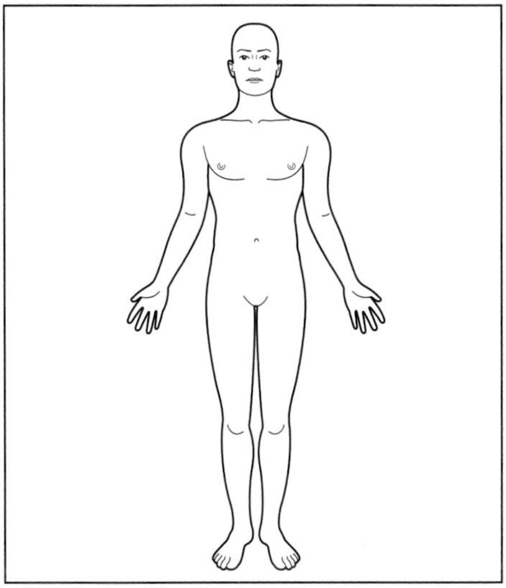

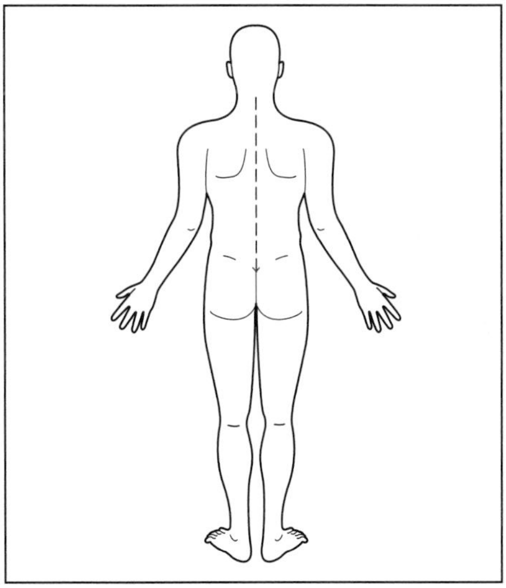

B

Figure 3.4, cont'd   (B) Pain chart for gathering descriptive terms from the patient, and for sketching pain patterns. (From Chaitow and Fritz 2006.)

pressure to lumbar muscles. After training, using bath-room scales, the students can usually apply precise amounts of pressure on request (Keating et al 1993).

Algometer

A basic algometer is a hand-held, spring-loaded, rubber-tipped, pressure-measuring device, that offers a means of achieving standardized pressure application. Using an algometer, sufficient pressure to produce pain is applied to preselected points, at a precise 90° angle to the skin. The measurement is taken when pain is reported.

An electronic version of this type of algometer allows recording of pressures applied, however these forms of algometer are used independently of actual treatment, to obtain feedback from the patient, to register the pressure being used when pain levels reach tolerance (see Fig. 3.5A,B).

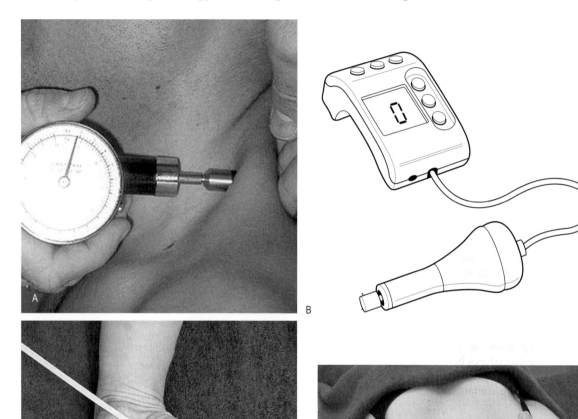

Figure 3.5   (A) Mechanical pressure algometer being used to measure applied pressure. (B) A version of an electronic algometer. (C) Electronic algometer pressure pad attached to thumb (and to computer). (D) Electronic algometer being used to evaluate pressure being applied to upper trapezius trigger point. (From Chaitow and Fritz 2006.)

A variety of other algometer designs exist, including a sophisticated version that is attached to the thumb or finger, with a lead running to an electronic sensor that is itself connected to a computer. This gives very precise readouts of the amount of pressure being applied by the finger or thumb during treatment (Fig. 3.5C,D)

Baldry (1993) suggests that algometers should be used to measure the degree of pressure required to produce symptoms, 'before and after deactivation of a trigger point, because when treatment is successful, the pressure threshold over the trigger point increases'.

If an algometer is not available, and in order to encourage only appropriate amounts of pressure being applied, it may be useful to practice simple palpation exercises such as those described below.

TISSUE 'LEVELS'

Palpation exercise

Pick (1999) has useful suggestions regarding the levels of tissue that you should try to reach by application of pressure, to be used in assessment and treatment. He describes the different levels of tissues you should be aiming for as follows.

Surface level
This is the first contact, molding to the contours of the structure, no actual pressure. This is just touching, without any pressure at all and is used to start treatment via the skin.

Working level
'The working level' is the level at which most manipulative procedures begin. Within this level, the practitioner can feel pliable counter-resistance to the applied force. The contact feels non-invasive and is usually well within the comfort zone of the subjects. Here the practitioner will find maximum control over the intracranial structures (Fig. 3.6).

Rejection levels
Pick suggests these levels are reached when tissue resistance is overcome, and discomfort/pain is reported. Rejection will occur at different degrees of pressure, in different areas and in different circumstances.

So how much pressure should be used?

1   *When working with the skin*: Surface level
2   *When palpating for trigger points*: Working level
3   *When testing for pain responses, and when treating trigger points*: Rejection level.

When you are at this rejection level, there is a feeling of the tissues pushing you away, you have to overcome the resistance to achieve a sustained compression.

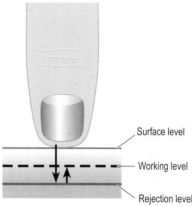

Figure 3.6   The concept of a 'working level'. Surface level involves touch without any pressure at all. Rejection level is where pressure meets a sense of the tissues 'pushing back' defensively. By reducing pressure slightly from the rejection level, the contact arrives at the working level, where perception of tissue change should be keenest, as well as there being an ability to distinguish normal from abnormal tissue (hypertonic, fibrotic, edematous, etc.) (After Dr Marc Pick DC 1999.) (From Chaitow 2005.)

KEY POINTS

- It is useful to have a record of the level of a patient's pain from the first visit, so that comparisons can be made over time
- There are variety of ways of achieving a record, ranging from simple questions and answers, to use of various scales and questionnaires
- The algometer (pressure gauge) is a tool that provides information as to how much pressure is needed to produce pain
- It is possible to develop sensitive palpation skills that allow a uniform amount of pressure to be used when testing the sensitivity of a patient, or a local point
- Information can and should be recorded so that progress (or no progress) can be measured accurately.

References

Baldry P 1993 Acupuncture, trigger points and musculoskeletal pain. Churchill Livingstone, Edinburgh

Chaitow L 2005 Cranial manipulation theory and practice, 2nd edn. Churchill Livingstone, Edinburgh

Chaitow L, DeLany J 2000 Clinical applications of neuromuscular technique, Volume 1. Churchill Livingstone, Edinburgh

Chaitow L, DeLany J 2002 Clinical applications of neuromuscular technique, Volume 2. Churchill Livingstone, Edinburgh

Chaitow L, Fritz S 2006 A massage therapist's guide to understanding, locating and treating myofascial trigger points. Churchill Livingstone, Edinburgh

Fryer G, Hodgson L 2005 The effect of manual pressure release on myofascial trigger points in the upper trapezius muscle. Journal of Bodywork and Movement Therapies (in press 2005)

Hong C-Z, Chen Y-N, Twehouse D, Hong D 1996 Pressure threshold for referred pain by compression on trigger point and adjacent area. Journal of Musculoskeletal Pain 4(3):61–79

Jensen M, Karoly P 1991 Control beliefs, coping efforts and adjustments to chronic pain. Journal of Consulting and Clinical Psychology 59:431–438

Keating J, Matyas T A, Bach T M et al 1993 The effect of training on physical therapists' ability to apply specific forces of palpation. Physical Therapy 73(1):45–53

Kelsey M 1951 Diagnosis of upper abdominal pain. Texas State Journal of Medicine 47:82–86

Kolt G, Andersen M 2004 Psychology in the physical and manual therapies. Churchill Livingstone, Edinburgh

Melzack R 1975 The McGill Pain Questionnaire: Major properties and scoring methods. Pain, 1, p 227–299.

Melzack R, Katz J 1999 Pain measurement in persons with pain. In: Wall P, Melzack R (eds) Textbook of pain, 4th edn. Churchill Livingstone, Edinburgh, p 409–420.

Nimmo R 1957 Receptors, effectors and tonus. Journal of the National Chiropractic Association 27(11):21

Nimmo R 1966 Workshop. British College of Naturopathy and Osteopathy, London

Oyama I, Rejba A, Lukban J et al 2004 Modified Thiele massage as therapeutic intervention for female patients with interstitial cystitis and high-tone pelvic floor dysfunction. Urology 64(5):862–865

Pick M 1999 Cranial sutures: analysis, morphology and manipulative strategies. Eastland Press, Seattle, p xx–xxi

Simons D, Travell J, Simons L 1999 Myofascial pain and dysfunction: the trigger point manual, Vol 1, Upper half of body, 2nd edn. Williams & Wilkins, Baltimore

Travell J, Simons D 1983 Myofascial pain and dysfunction: the trigger point manual, Vol 1, Upper body, 1st edn. Williams & Wilkins, Baltimore, p 671

Travell J, Simons D 1992 Myofascial pain and dysfunction: the trigger point manual, vol 2, the lower extremities. Williams and Wilkins, Baltimore

Weiss J 2001 Pelvic floor myofascial trigger points: manual therapy for interstitial cystitis and the urgency-frequency syndrome. Journal of Urology 166:2226–2231

Wolfe F, Ross K, Anderson J et al 1995 Aspects of fibromyalgia in the general population. Journal of Rheumatology 22:151–156

Chapter 4

Low back pain: palpation, observation and assessment approaches

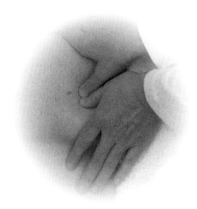

In this chapter, as explained in Chapter 1, we are not discussing those forms of back pain where pathology or structural anomalies are the causes (see Ch. 2).

The most common (97%) reported (Andersson 1997) 'causes' of low back pain (see Box 1.1) are:

- Heavy physical work
- Bending
- Twisting
- Lifting
- Pulling and pushing
- Repetitive work patterns
- Static postures
- Vibrations.

ADAPTATION

Almost all non-specific back pain arises from a background of failed adaptation. In order for the spine to remain flexible, stable and pain free, a number of basic requirements need to exist.

Liebenson (2000a) has pointed out, 'Spinal injury occurs when stress on a tissue exceeds the tissue's tolerance. It is not so much excessive load as too much motion which is the primary mechanism of injury. Spinal injury and recovery depends on a number of factors such as avoiding repetitive motion, end-range loading, and early morning spinal stress. Also important is improving muscular endurance'.

Canadian researcher, Stuart McGill (2004) describes the components that are required: 'The muscular and motor system must satisfy the requirements to sustain postures, create movements, brace against sudden motion or unexpected forces, build pressure, and assist challenged breathing, all the while ensuring sufficient stability'.

The lumbar spine, in particular, requires maximum stability and flexibility, if back pain and dysfunction are to be avoided.

MUSCLE FATIGUE

How tired muscles are is important. Fatigue is the end result of poor stamina, when muscles are unable to cope with whatever demands are being made.

Repetitive tasks such as bending and lifting gradually give way to stooping and decreased postural stability, as fatigue increases (Cholewicki et al 1997).

Liebenson (2000b) also emphasizes how important it is for the extensor muscles to have the quality of 'endurance', pointing out that the more easily fatigued the back muscles are, the more likely it is for back pain to commence.

THE KEY FEATURES NEEDED TO AVOID BACK PROBLEMS

Clearly, if the muscles of the back, pelvis and lower limbs are strong, balanced and supple, ligaments supply appropriate support to the joints, intervertebral discs are in good repair, and the motor supply to the soft tissues is optimal, most stress factors would be handled adequately, and no back pain would result from overuse and misuse.

But if some muscles are shortened, hypertonic and/or contain active trigger points, with other muscles inhibited and weak; or if neural input is less than optimal, and the normal firing sequence of muscles is uncoordinated, the load (bending, lifting, etc.) may easily overwhelm pelvic and spinal stabilizing efforts, allowing local injury to occur, with pain almost inevitably following.

There is then a failure of adaptation.

In order to offer appropriate care to a painful back, it is important to be able to evaluate shortness and weakness in those muscles involved in providing flexibility and stability, and to be able to identify trigger points in them.

QUESTIONS AND ANSWERS

The most important of these supportive contributory factors will be discussed in this chapter, as will some basic ways of assessing whether they are operating normally.

- Is this person's spine flexible and stable?
- Are the muscles that help to maintain stability and flexibility in good working order; toned, supple and free of local changes (such as trigger points) that could interfere with normal function?

Which structures are involved?

Paris (1997) has noted: 'In back management, … medical diagnosis is unable to find or agree on most causes of low back pain … the reason for this is that physicians are trained in disease, not in detecting dysfunctions, and dysfunctions are usually multiple rather than singular'.

Back pain seems to be largely caused by an accumulation of dysfunctions, each contributing a noxious stimulus, which, when a threshold is reached, are first interpreted as discomfort and eventually as pain, resulting in the patient seeking assistance.

Paris also suggests that we move away from single cause thinking, but instead try to decide on which structures are involved.

Awareness of the structures involved in back pain (muscle, joint, ligament, etc.), as well as the habits and/or events which have loaded (stressed) them, allows for the use of helpful prevention, therapeutic and rehabilitation interventions. This way of thinking is in line with research (Selye 1956) into stress that has shown that multiple minor stressors have the same effect as one major stress event (Fig. 4.1).

What are the 'minor' signs and features of dysfunction?

This message is of great value to us because it emphasizes the need to look for as many 'minor' signs and features of dysfunction as we can, by observation,

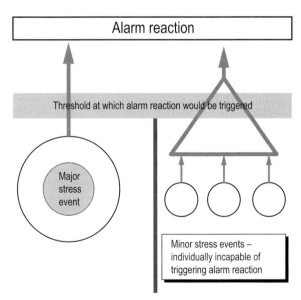

Figure 4.1 A combination of minor stresses, each incapable of triggering an alarm reaction in the general adaptation syndrome can, when combined or sustained, produce sufficient adaptive demand to initiate that alarm. In fibromyalgia a combination of major and minor biochemical, biomechanical and psychosocial stressors commonly seem to be simultaneously active. (From Chaitow 2003a.)

palpation and assessment, rather than seeking one single 'cause'.

- What's short?
- What's tight?
- What's contracted?
- What's restricted?
- What's weak?
- What's out of balance?
- What firing sequences are abnormal?
- What has happened, and/or what is the patient doing, to aggravate these changes?
- What can be done to help these changes to normalize?

Our task then is to reduce the adaptive burden that is making demands on the structures of the back and/or pelvis and, at the same time, to enhance the functional integrity of the back and pelvis so that the structures and tissues involved can better handle the abuses and misuses to which they are routinely subjected.

Soft tissue treatment methods, including massage and appropriate exercise, are major parts of the formula that will achieve the best therapeutic results.

FUNCTIONAL ASSESSMENTS

Janda (1982) and Lewit (1999) have developed a series of functional assessments that offer a quick and accurate 'snapshot' of how particular groups of muscles are behaving, and what this means in terms of their contribution to any pelvic or low back dysfunction.

There are three main functional assessments:

1 The prone hip extension test
2 The side-lying hip abduction test
3 Various strength tests, for example abdominal muscles and gluteals.

Hip extension test

- The patient lies prone and the therapist stands to the side, at waist level, with the cephalad hand spanning the lower lumbar musculature and assessing erector spinae activity, left and right (Fig. 4.2)
- The caudal hand is placed so that its heel lies on the gluteal muscle mass, with the fingertips resting on the hamstrings on the same side
- The person is asked to raise that leg into extension as the therapist assesses the firing sequence
- Which muscle fires (contracts) first?
- The normal activation sequence is (1) gluteus maximus, (2) hamstrings, followed by (3) contralateral erector spinae, and then (4) ipsilateral erector spinae
  Note: not all clinicians agree that this sequence is correct; some believe the hamstrings should fire first, or that there should be a simultaneous contraction of hamstrings and gluteus maximus, but all agree that the erector spinae should not contract first
- If the erectors on either side fire (contract) first, and take on the role of gluteus maximus as the prime

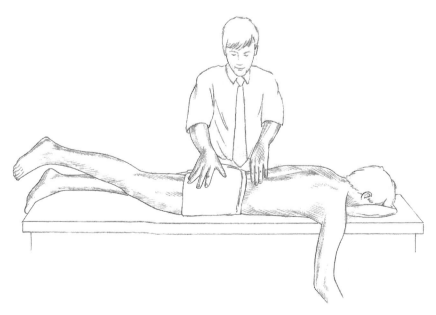

Figure 4.2 Hip extension test. The normal activation sequence is gluteus maximus, hamstrings, contralateral erector spinae, ipsilateral erector spinae.

movers in the task of extending the leg, they will become shortened and will further inhibit/weaken gluteus maximus

- Janda (1996) says, 'The poorest pattern occurs when the erector spinae on the ipsilateral side, or even the shoulder girdle muscles, initiate the movement and activation of gluteus maximus is weak and substantially delayed ... the leg lift is achieved by pelvic forward tilt and hyperlordosis of the lumbar spine, which undoubtedly stresses this region'.

The therapeutic approach   Stretch and normalize tone in the hamstrings and erector spinae muscles while suggesting exercises to help tone gluteus maximus (see Chs 7 and 8 in particular, for treatment details).

Hip abduction tests

1   Observation
- The patient lies on the side, ideally with head on a cushion, with the upper leg straight, in line with the trunk and the lower leg flexed at hip and knee, for balance
- You stand behind, at the level of the waist and observe (no hands-on yet) as your patient is asked to abduct the leg slowly
- Observe the area just above the crest of the pelvis – does it 'jump' at the outset of the abduction, or at least obviously activate before a 25° abduction has taken place? If so, the quadratus lumborum (QL) is overactive and probably short
- Have your patient relax completely and repeat the abduction which should be maintained for 10 s or so
- Does the leg 'drift' anteriorly during abduction? If so, the tensor fascia lata (TFL) is probably short
- Do the leg and foot turn outward (externally rotate)? If so, piriformis is probably short (Fig. 4.3A).

2   Palpation
- Now, still standing behind your side-lying patient, place one or two finger pads of your cephalad hand lightly on the tissues overlying quadratus lumborum, approximately 2 in (5 cm) lateral to the spinous process of L3 (Fig. 4.3B)
- Place your caudal hand so that the heel rests on gluteus medius and the finger pads on the TFL
- Assess the firing sequence of these muscles during hip abduction
- If the QL fires first (you will feel a strong twitch or 'jump' against your palpating fingers), it is overactive and short
- The ideal sequence is TFL followed by gluteus medius and finally QL (but not before about 20–25° abduction of the leg)

- If either TFL or QL are overactive (fire out of sequence), then they will have shortened, and the gluteus medius will be inhibited and weakened (Janda 1986).

The therapeutic approach   Stretch and lengthen the shortened muscles, and find ways for the patient to tone and strengthen the gluteus medius. Ideally, any trigger point activity that is adding to hypertonicity, or creating inhibition, should be identified and removed (see Chs 7 and 8 in particular, for treatment details).

Tests for muscle weakness

The most important muscles that influence spinal and pelvic stability, when they are inhibited/weak, are the gluteus maximus and medius, as well as the internal obliques and transversus abdominis (Hodges & Richardson 1996). These deep abdominal muscles are among the most important of the trunk's stabilizing muscles; their antagonists are the thoracolumbar erector spinae.

The transversus abdominis is the first and most used of these, being activated with almost every movement of the trunk, legs or arms (Hodges 1999). When the transversus is weak, the body may substitute the rectus abdominis, or the external oblique muscles, to do its work. When this happens, low back problems become more likely.

Trigger point activity in the abdominal or spinal muscles can inhibit the function of these muscles, as can excessive tightness/activity of the antagonists such as the erector spinae.

This following test screens for lumbopelvic instability during trunk flexion.

Test for weakness of internal obliques and transversus abdominis
- Your patient should lie supine, with the hips and knees flexed, and feet as close to the buttocks as possible with the arms folded across the chest
- You stand at the side of the table at the level of the patient's pelvis
- The patient is asked to raise the head and shoulders from the floor
- The feet should remain planted on the resting surface throughout the test, and not leave the table
- If the feet elevate off the supporting surface, this suggests recruitment of the hip flexors in order to provide adequate leverage to perform the task (Jull & Janda 1987)
- Does the abdomen 'dome', protrude, or does it flatten (Fig. 4.4A,B)?
- If the deeper stabilizing muscles, such as the transversus abdominis, are weak then they will not

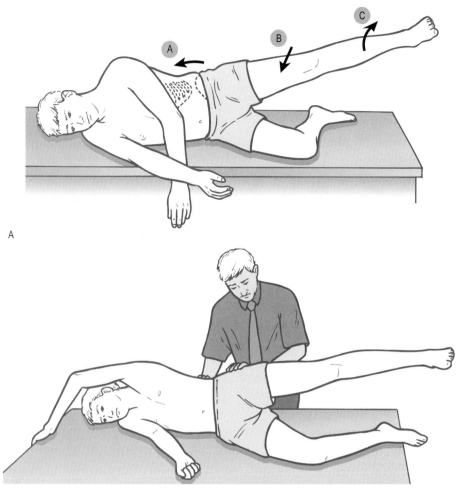

Figure 4.3   (A) Hip abduction observation test. Normal firing sequence is gluteus medius or tensor fascia lata (TFL) first and second, followed by quadratus lumborum (QL). If QL fires first it is overactive and will be short. If TFL is short, the leg will drift into flexion on abduction. If piriformis is short, the leg and foot will externally rotate during abduction. (B) Palpation assessment for quadratus lumborum overactivity. The muscle is palpated, as is the gluteus medius and TFL, during abduction of the leg. The correct firing sequence should be gluteus and TFL, followed at around 25° elevation by quadratus. If there is an immediate 'grabbing' action by quadratus it indicates overactivity, and therefore stress, so shortness can be assumed. (After Chaitow 2003.)

be able to hold the rectus abdominis down as it contracts, and it will dome
- Even if the head and shoulder can lift, without doming the abdomen, can that position be held for 10 s without difficulty (muscles start to quiver or shake)?
- The abdomen may dome, or the lower back may either stay straight or extend (bend backwards) rather than being able to round (flex) as the head and shoulders are lifted and the position is maintained
- This is even more likely to happen if the superficial abdominal muscles, such as the rectus abdominis, have lengthened as well as being weak (such as in

someone with a protruding 'pot' belly, see Crossed syndrome posture below).

The therapeutic approach   If weakness is demonstrated in these core stabilizing muscles, there is an urgency to initiate toning exercises as described in Chapter 8. In addition, reasons for the weakness should be addressed, including improved posture, and removal of excessive tone and shortening in the antagonists, such as erector spinae and hip flexors. Ideally, any trigger point activity that may be adding to hypertonicity, or creating inhibition, should be identified and removed (see also Ch. 7).

Test for weakness of the gluteus medius

Method 1 (Lee 1997)

- The patient should be side-lying, with the leg to be tested uppermost and knee extended
- The hip is placed and supported in slight extension, abduction and external rotation, and the patient is

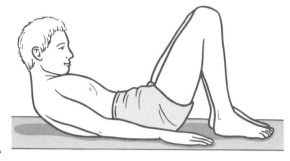

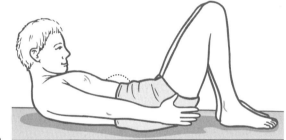

A

B

Figure 4.4 (A,B) Test position to assess internal oblique and transversus abdominis strength. (After Chaitow 2003b.)

asked to maintain the position of the trunk and leg when support for the leg is released (Fig. 4.5)

- When the support is released, and if the gluteus medius is weak, there may be posterior pelvic rotation if TFL assists the effort; or the spine may be pulled into side-flexion as quadratus attempts to brace the leg
- If the patient can maintain the original position for 10 s, pressure is then applied to the leg in the direction of hip flexion, adduction and internal rotation, thereby resisting gluteus medius posterior fibers
- If the posterior fibers of gluteus medius are weak, the patient will be unable to hold the position against pressure.

If weakness is established, there are negative implications for the sacroiliac joint during the gait cycle.

The therapeutic approach Reasons for the relative weakness should be assessed, which could possibly involve excess tone in the antagonists, or trigger points in gluteus medius or associated muscles. Special attention should be given to searching for trigger points in those muscles which refer into the gluteus medius region, such as the quadratus lumborum, gluteus maximus and minimus, iliocostalis lumborum, piriformis, and rectus abdominis (see Chs 7 and 8 for treatment details).

Method 2

- For this test (known as the Trendelenburg test) the patient stands and the sacral dimples (which should

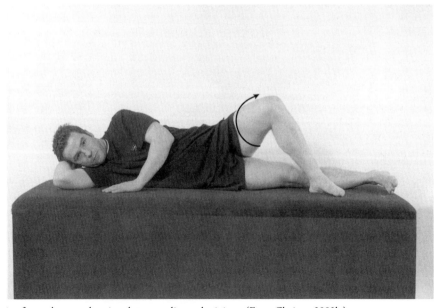

Figure 4.5 Testing for weakness and toning gluteus medius and minimus (From Chaitow 2003b.)

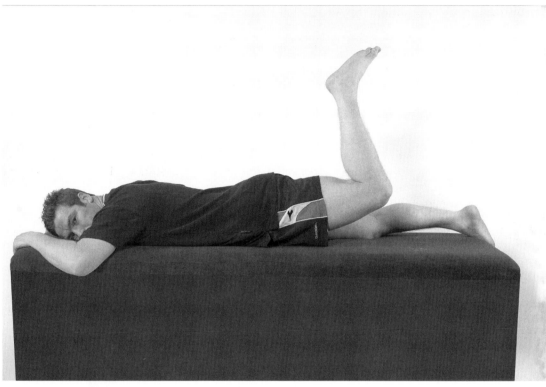

Figure 4.6 Test and toning position for gluteus maximus. (From Chaitow 2003b.)

be level) are located, and their relative height to each other noted
- The patient stands on one leg (say the right) and the gluteus medius on the right side should contract, sidebending the pelvis to the right, causing elevation of the pelvis on the left
- If this happens, the test is negative (i.e. the muscle is behaving normally)
- If the muscle is inadequate to the task of side-bending the pelvis (i.e. it stays level or the left side drops), the test is positive and gluteus medius is assumed to be weak or not functioning normally, on the right (Fig. 5.16).

The therapeutic approach The reasons for this dysfunction should be investigated and might include pathologies which bring the attachments close to each other (fractures of the greater trochanter, slipped capital femoral epiphysis), congenital dislocation, poliomyelitis, or nerve root lesions (Hoppenfeld 1976). Referral to a practitioner licensed to make a diagnosis is suggested.

Test for weakness of the gluteus maximus
- The patient lies prone
- The knee on the side to be tested is flexed to 90°

- The thigh is lifted without arching the back and this position is held until the task becomes difficult (Fig. 4.6)
- If the position cannot be held for 10 s, this suggests weakness of the gluteus maximus
- If the position can be held without difficulty for 20 s, this suggests normal strength in gluteus maximus
- If the indication is of weakness, psoas may be shortened and hypertonic.

The therapeutic approach Remove overactivity in antagonists (such as psoas) and increase tone in the weakened gluteus maximus muscle (possibly by regularly adopting the test position until maintaining the contraction for 20 s becomes easy). Ideally, any trigger point activity adding to hypertonicity, or creating inhibition, should be identified and removed (see Chs 7 and 8 for treatment details).

When the gluteus maximus is weakened Lee (1997) provides an insight into the problems that can occur when the gluteus maximus is weakened: 'Clinically gluteus maximus appears to become inhibited whenever the sacroiliac joint (SIJ) is irritated or in dysfunction. The consequences to gait can be catastrophic when … the stride length shortens, and the hamstrings are overused to compensate for the loss of hip extensor power ... in time, the SIJ can become hypermobile. This is often seen in athletes with repetitive hamstring strains. The hamstrings remain overused and vulnerable to intramuscular tears'.

The therapeutic approach should be to normalize the strength of the gluteals and to reduce the hypertonicity of the hamstrings.

Tests for spinal muscle (e.g. multifidi) weakness
When there is low back pain, a major influence is often found via the multifidi (Liebenson 2000b).

These muscles may actually atrophy when unused, as happens when – because of back pain – a person rests instead of starting some form of rehabilitation exercising as soon as the acute phase has eased. This is known as 'deconditioning' and the exercises described in Chapter 8 can help to prevent this.

Standing arm elevation test for multifidi weakness
- The patient stands against a wall, with the buttocks and spine touching the wall, and the heels placed about 2 in (5 cm) from it
- The arms should be raised directly in front so that the backs of your hands can be placed against the wall above the head (Fig. 4.7).

If, as this is done, the low back arches forward, or the wall cannot be touched by the backs of the hands, the suggestion is that the mid-spine (mid-thoracic) is restricted and that there is a need for mobilization of that area, as well as improvement of stability of the deep muscles such as multifidi (see exercise description below).

Trunk extension test and exercise
- The patient lies on the floor prone, with hands interlocked behind the neck, elbows pointing forward so that they lie as close to parallel with the floor as possible
- The chest is lifted from the floor approximately 2 in (5 cm) before lying down again. Figure 4.8A,B shows examples of correct and incorrect performance
- The legs and feet should remain in touch with the floor throughout (there will be a tendency for the feet and lower legs to rise, and this shows excessive effort from the superficial erector spinae)
- With a pause of no more than 2 s between each repetition, this movement should be repeated 15 times, with the final lift being held for 30 s.

If the patient accomplishes this, the multifidi are normal. If not, this exercise can be repeated until it is easily accomplished.

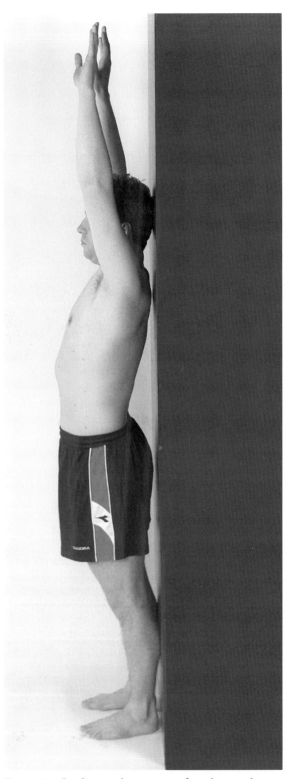

Figure 4.7 Standing arm elevation test performed incorrectly: arms cannot reach wall and low back arches. (From Chaitow 2003b.)

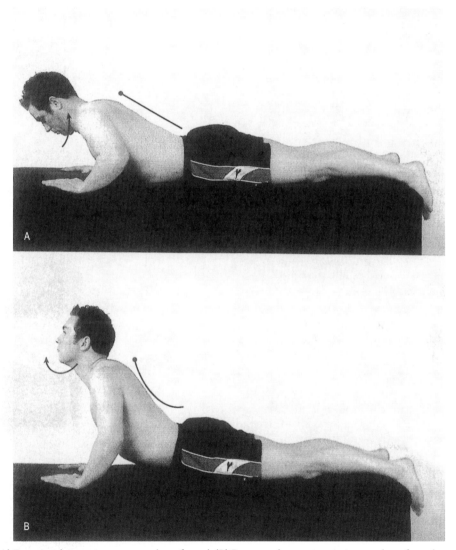

Figure 4.8 (A) Prone trunk extension test correctly performed. (B) Prone trunk extension test incorrectly performed: note neck and spine extend instead of staying in line. (From Chaitow 2003b.) Note: The method illustrated is a less stressful version than the one described, where hands are clasped behind the neck.

CROSSED SYNDROME PATTERNS

As compensation occurs to overuse, misuse and disuse of muscles of the spine and pelvis, some muscles become overworked, shortened and restricted, with others becoming inhibited and weak, and body-wide postural changes take place that have been characterized as 'crossed syndromes' (Lewit 1999) (Fig. 4.9A,B). These crossed patterns demonstrate the imbalances that occur as antagonists become inhibited due to the overactivity of specific postural muscles. The effect on spinal and pelvic mechanics of these imbalances (which would have shown up when the hip extension and hip abduction tests were performed) would be to create an environment in which pain and dysfunction (such as sacroiliac joint) would become more likely to occur.

One of the main tasks in rehabilitation of such pain and dysfunction is to normalize these imbalances, to release and stretch whatever is over-short and tight, and to encourage tone in those muscles that have become inhibited and weakened (Liebenson 1996).

- In the upper crossed pattern, we see how the deep neck flexors and the lower fixators of the shoulder (serratus anterior, lower and middle trapezius) have weakened (and possibly lengthened), while their antagonists the upper trapezius, levator scapula and the pectorals will have shortened and tightened
- Also short and tight, are the cervical extensor muscles, the suboccipitals, and the rotator cuff muscles of the shoulder
- In the lower crossed pattern we see, in Figure 4.9B, that the abdominal muscles have weakened, as have the gluteals, and at the same time psoas and erector spinae will have shortened and tightened
- Also short and tight, are tensor fascia lata, piriformis, quadratus lumborum, hamstrings and latissimus dorsi.

In the section below outlining tests for shortness, the key muscles that have influence on the low back and pelvis are listed (see Chs 7 and 8 for treatment options).

Tests for muscle shortness

The tests for muscle shortness, listed below, focus on those most likely to be involved in both back and pelvic pain problems. In Chapter 5, which pays specific attention to pelvic pain, additional assessments will be described. The following tests are derived from the work of Janda (1983), Kendall et al (1993) and a variety of other sources.

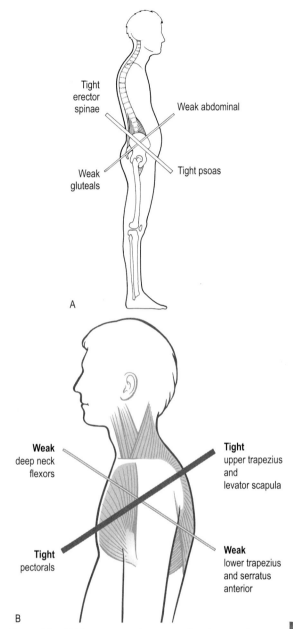

Figure 4.9 (A) Lower crossed patterns of weakness and tightness. (B) Upper crossed patterns of weakness and tightness. (From Chaitow 2003b.)

Test for hamstring shortness: upper fibers (straight leg raise)
- In order to assess for shortened hamstrings (biceps, femoris, semitendinosus and semimembranosus), your patient should lie supine with the leg to be tested outstretched and the other leg flexed at both knee and hip, to relax the low back

- In order to assess tightness in the left leg hamstrings (upper fibers), you should be standing at the side of the leg to be tested, facing the head of the table
- The lower leg is supported by your caudal hand, keeping the knee of that leg in light extension and if possible resting the heel of that leg in the bend of the elbow to prevent lateral rotation
- The cephalad hand can then rest on the hamstrings, around mid-thigh, to evaluate for 'bind' as elevation takes place (Fig. 4.10A)
- The range of movement into hip flexion should (with a supple hamstring group, and no neural restrictions) allow painless elevation of the tested leg to about 80° before tension is noted
- Does the first sign of resistance, bind, occur before 80°?
- If so, the hamstrings are almost certainly shortened.

The therapeutic approach   Aim at releasing and relaxing, and possibly stretching, the shortened hamstring fibers (see Chs 7 and 8 for treatment details).

Test for hamstring shortness: lower fibers
- To make this assessment, the tested leg is taken into full hip flexion (helped by the patient holding the upper thigh with both hands) (Fig. 4.10B)
- You should place a hand onto the fibers just inferior to the popliteal space to assess for bind as the leg straightens
- The knee is then passively straightened until resistance is felt, or bind is noted by this palpation hand resting on the lower hamstrings
- If the knee cannot easily straighten with the hip flexed, this indicates shortness in the lower hamstring fibers, and a degree of pull behind the knee and lower thigh will be reported during any attempt to straighten the leg
- If the knee is capable of being straightened with the hip flexed, having previously not been capable of achieving an 80°, straight-leg raise, then the lower fibers are cleared of shortness, and it is the upper hamstring fibers which require therapeutic attention.

The therapeutic approach   Aim at releasing and relaxing, and possibly stretching, the shortened hamstrings (see Chs 7 and 8 for treatment details).

Caution   In a person with a history of an unstable sacroiliac joint, or in someone who is generally hypermobile, it is possible that excessive tension in the hamstrings (and/or the presence in these muscles of active trigger points) could be acting to stabilize the joint via traction on the sacrotuberous ligament

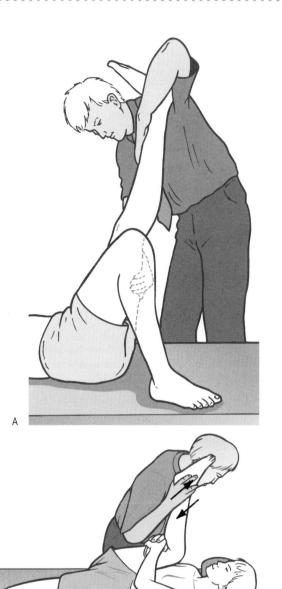

A

B

Figure 4.10   (A) Assessment for shortness of hamstring, upper fibers, by palpation during leg raising. (After Chaitow 2003c.) (B) Assessment for shortness of hamstring, lower fibers, by palpation during leg straightening. (From Chaitow 2003c.)

(Vleeming et al 1997). In such cases, caution should be employed before stretching the hamstrings, or deactivating the trigger points, as the joint could be made more unstable.

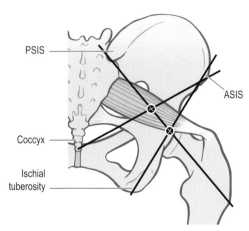

Figure 4.11   Landmarks are used as coordinates to locate the attachment of piriformis at the hip, and also the site of major trigger point activity in the belly of the muscle. (From Chaitow 2003c.)

Palpating for shortness of piriformis
When short, the piriformis will cause the affected side leg of the supine individual to appear to be short and externally rotated.

- Have your patient side-lying, tested side uppermost
- You should stand in front of and facing the pelvis
- In order to contact the insertion of piriformis, draw two imaginary lines: one runs from the ASIS to the ischial tuberosity and the other from the PSIS to the most prominent point of the trochanter (Fig. 4.11)
- Where these lines cross, just posterior to the trochanter, is the attachment of the muscle, and pressure here will produce marked discomfort if piriformis is short or irritated
- In order to locate the most common trigger point site, in the belly of the muscle, the line from the ASIS should be taken to the tip of the coccyx rather than the ischial tuberosity
- The other line from the PSIS to the trochanter prominence is the same as above
- Pressure where one line crosses the other will access the mid-point of the belly of piriformis, where trigger points are common
- Light compression here, that produces a painful response ('jump sign'), is indicative of a stressed and probably shortened muscle.

The therapeutic approach   Aim at releasing and relaxing, and possibly stretching, the shortened piriformis fibers (see Chs 7 and 8 for treatment details).

Paravertebral muscle shortness assessment
1   Your patient should be seated on the treatment table, legs extended, pelvis vertical.

- Flexion is introduced in order to approximate the forehead to the knees without strain
- An even curve should be observed and a distance of about 10 cm from the knees achieved by the forehead
- No knee flexion should occur and the movement should be a spinal one, not involving pelvic tilting (Fig. 4.12)
2   Your patient should be seated at the edge of the table, knees flexed and lower legs hanging over the edge, relaxing the hamstrings.
- Forward bending is introduced so that the forehead approximates the knees
- If flexion of the trunk is greater in this position than when the legs were straight, then there is probably tilting of the pelvis and shortened hamstring involvement
3   Observe the spinal curve as your patient sits in the forward bending position, as in 1, above.
- During these assessments, there should be a uniform degree of flexion throughout the spine, with a 'C' curve apparent when looked at from the side
- However, all too commonly, areas of shortening in the spinal muscles may be observed, particularly as areas which are 'flat', where little or no flexion is taking place
- In some instances lordosis may be maintained in the lumbar spine even on full flexion, or flexion may be very limited, even without such lordosis
- There may also be obvious overstretching of the upper back, as compensation for the relative tightness of the lower back
- Generally 'flat' areas of the spine indicate local shortening of the erector spinae group
- Can you observe 'flat', tense, areas of the spine, during any of these flexion exercises?
- Identify such areas and palpate them lightly as your patient moves into flexion
- Compare the feel of the tissues as they tighten, bind, compared with those areas which are flexible, where the curve is normal
- Also, if you identify flat areas, have your patient lie prone and palpate lightly with your fingertips to assess the degree of hypertonicity.

See which of the following variables is evident in your patient:

1   Normal length of erector spinae muscles and posterior thigh muscles
2   Tight gastrocnemius and soleus; an inability to dorsiflex the feet indicates tightness of the plantar-flexor group

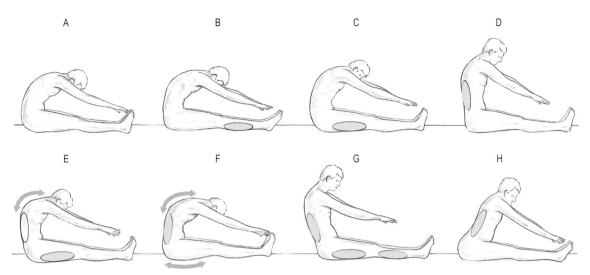

Figure 4.12   Tests for shortness of the erector spinae and associated postural muscles. (A) Normal length of erector spinae muscles and posterior thigh muscles. (B) Tight gastrocnemius and soleus; the inability to dorsiflex the feet indicates tightness of the plantarflexor group. (C) Tight hamstring muscles, which cause the pelvis to tilt posteriorly. (D) Tight low back erector spinae muscles. (E) Tight hamstring; slightly tight low back muscles and overstretched upper back muscles. (F) Slightly shortened lower back muscles, stretched upper back muscles and slightly stretched hamstrings. (G) Tight low back muscles, hamstrings and gastrocnemius/soleus. (H) Very tight low back muscles, with lordosis maintained even in flexion. (From Chaitow 2003c.)

3   Tight hamstring muscles, which cause the pelvis to tilt posteriorly
4   Tight low back erector spinae muscles
5   Tight hamstring; slightly tight lower back muscles and overstretched upper back muscles
6   Slightly shortened lower back muscles, stretched upper back muscles and slightly stretched hamstrings
7   Tight lower back muscles, hamstrings and gastrocnemius/soleus
8   Very tight low back muscles, with lordosis maintained even in flexion.

The therapeutic approach   Aim towards restoring normal flexion potential to the spine by means of releasing and relaxing excessively short and tight muscles and encouraging better tone in weakened ones (see Chs 7 and 8 for treatment details).

Breathing wave
With the patient prone, observation is made of the 'breathing wave' – the movement of the spine from sacrum to base of neck on deep inhalation.

A full inhalation in this position, with a fully flexible spine, will demonstrate a wave-like movement starting close to the sacrum and finishing in the upper back.

When areas of the spine are restricted (and this would have shown up in the seated flexion obser-

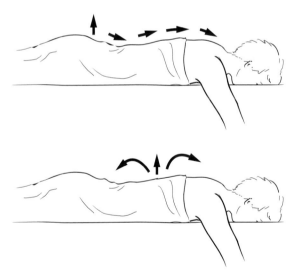

Figure 4.13   Functional (top) and dysfunctional (bottom) breathing wave movement patterns. (Reproduced with kind permission from Chaitow & DeLany 2000).

vation discussed above, particularly in examples 4, 5, 6 and 7) the spinal response to inhalation will be of several segments rising together as a 'block' (Fig. 4.13).

Pain is common in the more mobile segments of the spine, immediately above and below such restricted areas, and this may reduce or vanish when mobility is restored.

The therapeutic approach   It is these 'blocked' areas of the spine that need to be gently mobilized by means of releasing and relaxing of associated muscles, as well as by stretching exercises (see Chs 7 and 8 for treatment details).

Breathing pattern and spinal well-being
Motor control is a key component in spinal (and all joint) injury prevention. Loss of motor control involves failure to control joints, commonly because of poor coordination of the agonist-antagonist muscle co-activation.

Three subsystems work together to maintain spinal stability (Panjabi 1992):

- The central nervous subsystem (control)
- The osteoligamentous subsystem (passive)
- The muscle subsystem (active).

There is evidence that the effects of breathing pattern disorders, such as hyperventilation, result in a variety of negative influences and interferences, capable of modifying each of these three subsystems (Chaitow 2004).

- Breathing pattern disorders (the extreme form of which is hyperventilation) automatically increase levels of anxiety and apprehension, which may be sufficient to alter motor control and to markedly influence balance control (Balaban & Thayer 2001).
- Hyperventilation results in respiratory alkalosis, leading to reduced oxygenation of tissues (including the brain), smooth muscle constriction, heightened pain perception, speeding up of spinal reflexes, increased excitability of the corticospinal system (Macefield & Burke 1991, Seyal et al 1998), hyper-irritability of motor and sensory axons (Mogyoros et al 1997), changes in serum calcium and magnesium levels (George 1964) and encouragement of the development of myofascial trigger points (Simons et al 1999) – all or any of which, in one way or another, are capable of modifying normal motor control of skeletal musculature.
- Diaphragmatic and transversus abdominis tone are key features in provision of core stability, however it has been noted that reduction in the support offered to the spine, by the muscles of the torso, may occur if there is a load challenge to the low back combined with a breathing challenge (McGill et al 1995).
- It has been demonstrated that, after approximately 60 s of over-breathing, the postural (tonic) and phasic

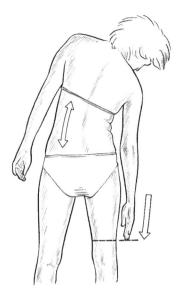

Figure 4.14   MET self-treatment for quadratus lumborum. Patient assesses range of sidebending to the right. (From Chaitow 2001.)

functions of both the diaphragm and transversus abdominis are reduced or absent (Hodges et al 2001).

It is therefore important to pay attention to the breathing pattern of anyone with back pain, and guidelines are offered in Chapter 8.

Quadratus lumborum muscle shortness assessment
The hip abduction test (above) will have given a clear indication of overactivity of QL, and the simple assessment (below) identifies the shorter side, as well as the degree of shortness (Fig. 4.14).

- The patient stands with back towards you
- Place your index fingers onto the crests of the pelvis, left and right and evaluate whether they are level or not
- Any leg length disparity (based on pelvic crest height) should be equalized by using a book or pad under the short leg heel
- With the patient's feet shoulder-width apart, a pure side-bending is requested, so that the patient runs a hand down the lateral thigh/calf. (Normal level of side-bending excursion allows the fingertips to reach to just below the knee.)
- If sidebending to one side is less than to the other, then QL is apparently short on the side away from which the excursion is shortest

- If there is an obvious shortness *and* the short side was also shown to be overactive during the hip abduction test, then treatment of the QL is called for.

This is outlined in Chapters 7 and 8.

Rectus femoris, iliopsoas muscle shortness assessment
- The patient lies supine with buttocks (coccyx) as close to the end of the table as possible, the non-tested leg in flexion at both hip and knee, held by the patient
- Full flexion of the hip helps to maintain the pelvis in full rotation with the lumbar spine flat. This is essential if the test is to be meaningful and stress on the spine avoided
- If the thigh of the tested leg lies in a horizontal position in which it is parallel to the floor/table (Fig. 4.15A) then the indication is that iliopsoas is not short
- If however, the thigh rises above the horizontal (Fig. 4.15B) then iliopsoas is probably short
- In this supine testing position, if the lower leg of the tested side fails to hang down to an almost 90° angle with the thigh, vertical to the floor, then shortness of rectus femoris is indicated (Fig. 4.15B)
- Rectus femoris shortness can be confirmed by seeing whether or not the heel on the tested side can easily flex to touch the buttock when the patient is prone. If rectus femoris is short, the heel will not easily reach the buttock (Fig. 4.16).
- If TFL is short (a further test proves it, see below) then there should be an obvious groove apparent on the lateral thigh, and sometimes the whole lower leg will deviate laterally

Treatment choices are outlined in Chapters 7 and 8.

Tensor fascia lata muscle shortness assessment
- The test is a modified form of Ober's test
- The patient is side-lying with back close to the edge of the table
- You stand behind the patient, whose lower leg is flexed at hip and knee and held in this position, by the patient, for stability
- You support the leg to be tested as illustrated in Figure 4.17
- You should ensure that there is no hip flexion, which would nullify the test
- The leg is extended to the position where the iliotibial band lies over the greater trochanter
- The tested leg is supported at ankle and knee, with the whole leg in its anatomical position, neither abducted nor adducted, and not forward or backward of the trunk
- You should carefully introduce flexion at the knee to 90°, without allowing the hip to flex, and then,

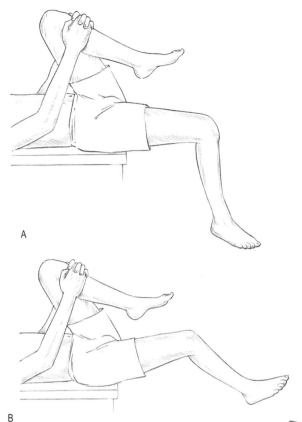

A

B

Figure 4.15 (A) Test position for shortness of hip flexors. Note that the hip on the non-tested side must be fully flexed to produce full pelvic rotation. The position shown is normal. (B) In the test position, if the thigh is elevated (i.e. not parallel with the table) probable psoas shortness is indicated. The inability of the lower leg to hang more or less vertically towards the floor indicates probable rectus femoris shortness (TFL shortness can produce a similar effect). (From Chaitow 2001.)

while supporting the limb at the ankle, remove your hand from under the knee and allow it to fall towards the table
- If the TFL is normal, the thigh and knee will fall easily, with the knee usually contacting the table surface (unless there is unusual hip width, or a short thigh length preventing this)
- If the upper leg remains aloft, with little sign of 'falling' towards the table, then either the patient is not relaxing, or the TFL is short and does not allow it to fall
- As a rule, the band will palpate as tender under such conditions.

Treatment options are outlined in Chapters 7 and 8.

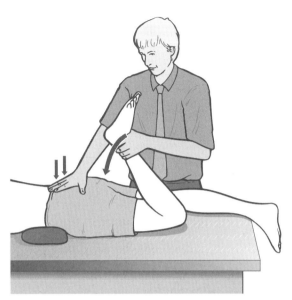

Figure 4.16 Test for rectus femoris shortness. A normal muscle will allow the heel to reach the buttock without force. (From Chaitow 2001.)

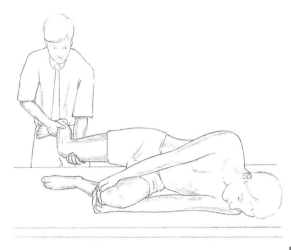

Figure 4.17 Assessment for shortness of TFL – modified Ober's test. When the hand supporting the flexed knee is removed the thigh should fall to the table if TFL is not short. (From Chaitow 2001.)

PALPATING FOR TRIGGER POINTS

In osteopathic medicine, an acronym 'STAR' is used as a reminder of the characteristics of somatic dysfunction, such as myofascial trigger points.

STAR stands for:

- **S**ensitivity (or 'tenderness'): this is the one feature that is almost always present when there is soft tissue dysfunction
- **T**issue texture change: the tissues usually 'feel' different (for example they may be tense, fibrous, swollen, hot, cold or have other 'differences' from normal)
- **A**symmetry: there will commonly be an imbalance on one side, compared with the other, but this is not always the case
- **R**ange of motion reduced: muscles will probably not be able to reach their normal resting length, or joints may have a restricted range.

If two or three of these features are present, this is enough to confirm that there is a problem, a dysfunction. It does not however explain why the problem exists, but is a start in the process towards understanding the patient's symptoms.

Research (Fryer et al 2004) has confirmed that this traditional osteopathic palpation method is valid. When tissues in the thoracic paraspinal muscles were found to be 'abnormal' (tense, dense, indurated), the same tissues (using an algometer; see Ch. 3) were also found to have a lowered pain threshold. Less pressure was needed to create pain.

While the 'tenderness', altered texture and range of motion characteristics, as listed in the STAR acronym, are always true for trigger points, additional trigger point changes have been listed by Simons and colleagues (1999):

- The soft tissues housing the trigger point will demonstrate a painful limit to stretch range of motion, whether the stretching is active, or passive (i.e. the patient is stretching the muscle, or you are stretching the muscle)
- In such muscles, there is usually pain or discomfort when it is contracted against resistance, with no movement taking place (i.e. an isometric contraction)
- The amount of force the muscle can generate is reduced when it contains active (or latent) trigger points; it is weaker than a normal muscle
- A palpable taut band, with an exquisitely tender nodule exists, and this should be found by palpation, unless the trigger lies in very deep muscle and is not accessible
- Pressure on the tender spot produces pain familiar to the patient, and often a pain response ('jump sign').

Treatment of trigger points is outlined and discussed in Chapters 7 and 8.

KEY POINTS

- There are usually a number of 'causes' and aggravating factors, as well as different structures, involved in any case of back pain, rather than just one cause
- The first objectives are to identify what these factors and tissues are, and to use treatment to enhance function and reduce the adaptive load
- Functional tests (hip abduction for example) demonstrate through observation and palpation which muscles are being overused, misused or disused and are therefore likely to be shortened and/or weakened
- These patterns of imbalance create crossed syndromes that can be recognized by observation
- Tests for weakness indicate which muscles require toning; either through exercise, or through removal of inhibition from antagonists, or both
- Tests for shortness indicate which muscles require releasing, relaxing and stretching

- Palpation methods using the STAR ingredients offer a useful way of identifying local dysfunction
- Tests for the presence of trigger points help to locate and identify those in need of deactivation (active points)
- Breathing pattern disorders can disturb motor control of the spine and encourage back problems
- By restoring balanced muscle activity, reducing tightness, increasing tone in weak structures, encouraging better breathing, and deactivating trigger points – normal function is encouraged. Stages of care should include:
  - Relieving pain (massage, trigger point deactivation, ice, etc.)
  - Easing adaptive demands (better posture and use patterns)
  - Improving function (exercise, improved stability etc.)

References

Andersson G 1997 Epidemiology of spinal disorders. In: Frymoyer JL (ed.) The adult spine, 2nd edition. Raven Press, New York, p 93–141

Balaban C, Thayer J 2001 Neurological bases for balance-anxiety links. Journal of Anxiety Disorders 15(1–2):53–79

Chaitow L 2001 Muscle energy techniques, 2nd edn. Churchill Livingstone, Edinburgh

Chaitow L 2003a Fibromyalgia syndrome, 2nd edn. Churchill Livingstone, Edinburgh

Chaitow L 2003b Maintaining body balance, flexibility and stability. Churchill Livingstone, Edinburgh

Chaitow L 2003c Palpation skills. Churchill Livingstone, Edinburgh

Chaitow L 2004 Breathing pattern disorders, motor control, and low back pain. Journal of Osteopathic Medicine 7(1):34–41

Chaitow L, DeLany J 2000 Clinical applications of neuromuscular technique, Volume 1. Churchill Livingstone, Edinburgh

Chaitow L, Bradley D, Gilbert C 2002 Multidisciplinary approaches to breathing pattern disorders. Churchill Livingstone, Edinburgh

Cholewicki J, Panjabi M, Khachatryan A 1997 Stabilizing function of the trunk flexor-extensor muscles around a neutral spine posture. Spine 19:2207–2212

Fryer G, Morris T, Gibbons P 2004 Relation between thoracic paraspinal tissues and pressure sensitivity measured by digital algometer. Journal of Osteopathic Medicine 7(2):64–69

George S 1964 Changes in serum calcium, serum phosphate and red cell phosphate during hyperventilation. New England Journal of Medicine 270:726–728

Hodges P 1999 Is there a role for transversus abdominis in lumbo-pelvic stability? Manual Therapy 4(2):74–86

Hodges P, Heinjnen I, Gandevia S 2001 Postural activity of the diaphragm is reduced in humans when respiratory demand increases. Journal of Physiology 537(3):999–1008

Hodges P, Richardson C 1996 Inefficient muscular stabilization of the lumbar spine associated with low back pain. Spine 21:2640–2650

Hoppenfeld S 1976 Physical examination of the spine and extremities. Appleton and Lange, Norwalk

Janda V 1982 Introduction to functional pathology of the motor system. Proceedings of the VIIth Commonwealth and International Conference on Sport. Physiotherapy in Sport 3:39

Janda V 1983 Muscle function testing. Butterworths, London

Janda V 1986 Muscle weakness and inhibition (pseudoparesis) in back pain syndromes. In: Grieve G (ed.) Modern manual therapy of the vertebral column. Churchill Livingstone, Edinburgh

Janda V 1996 Evaluation of muscular imbalance. In: Liebenson C (ed.) Rehabilitation of the spine. Williams and Wilkins, Baltimore

Jull G, Janda V 1987 Muscles and motor control in low back pain: Assessment and management. In: Twomey L, Grieve G (eds) Physical therapy of the low back. Churchill Livingstone, Edinburgh, p 253–278

Kendall F, McCreary E, Provance P 1993 Muscles, testing and function, 4th edn. Williams & Wilkins, Baltimore

Lee D 1997 Treatment of pelvic instability. In: Vleeming A, Mooney V, Dorman T et al (eds) Movement, stability and low back pain. Churchill Livingstone, Edinburgh

Lewit K 1999 Chain reactions in the locomotor system. Journal of Orthopaedic Medicine 21:52–58

Lewit K 1999 Manipulation in rehabilitation of the motor system, 3rd edn. Butterworth Heinemann, London

Liebenson C 1996 Rehabilitation of the spine. Williams & Wilkins, Baltimore

Liebenson C 2000a The quadratus lumborum and spinal stability. Journal of Bodywork and Movement Therapies 4(1):49–54

Liebenson C 2000b The trunk extensors and spinal stability. Journal of Bodywork and Movement Therapies 4(4):246–249

Macefield G, Burke D 1991 Paresthesia and tetany induced by voluntary hyperventilation. Brain 114:527–540

McGill S 2004 Functional anatomy of lumbar stability. Proceedings of the 5th Interdisciplinary World Congress on Low Back and Pelvic Pain. Melbourne, Australia, p 3–9

McGill S, Sharratt M, Seguin J 1995 Loads on spinal tissues during simultaneous lifting and ventilatory challenge. Ergonomics 38(9):1772–1792

Mogyoros I, Kiernan K, Burke D et al 1997 Excitability changes in human sensory and motor axons during hyperventilation and ischaemia. Brain 120(2):317–325

Panjabi M 1992 The stabilizing system of the spine. Part 1. Function, dysfunction, adaptation, and enhancement. Journal of Spinal Disorders 5:383–389

Paris S 1997 Differential diagnosis of lumbar and pelvic pain. In: Vleeming A, Mooney V, Dorman T et al (eds) Movement, stability and low back pain. Churchill Livingstone, New York

Selye H 1956 The stress of life. McGraw Hill, New York

Seyal M, Mull B, Gage B 1998 Increased excitability of the human corticospinal system with hyperventilation. Electroencephalography and Clinical Neurophysiology/Electromyography and Motor Control 109(3):263–267

Simons D, Travell J, Simons L 1999 Myofascial pain and dysfunction: the trigger point manual, Vol 1, Upper half of body, 2nd edn. Williams & Wilkins, Baltimore

Vleeming A, Mooney V, Dorman T et al (eds) 1997 Movement, stability and low back pain. Churchill Livingstone, Edinburgh

Chapter 5

Pelvic pain

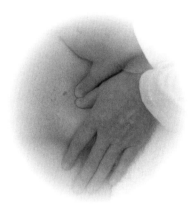

The reason for creating two chapters instead of one focused on low back pain and pelvic pain is in order to separate those aspects of assessment that relate particularly to pelvic, sacral, sacroiliac and iliosacral symptoms, in contrast to pain deriving specifically from spinal structures.

In reality of course, a restricted sacroiliac joint (SIJ), or a torsioned sacrum, will produce a situation in which spinal tissues and joints will become distressed, and probably painful – just as a restricted segment in the lumbar spine can cause adaptive demands and distress to the sacroiliac joints. So pain in the pelvis and pain in the spine are capable of feeding into each other.

It is also clear that patterns of pain caused by trigger points in the lower abdomen can refer symptoms into the back and/or the pelvic structures (see Fig. 3.1).

From the perspective of a massage therapist, it is important to be able to identify SIJ and other pelvic dysfunctions, because, in some instances, appropriate soft tissue treatment will be able to reduce or normalize the dysfunctional state.

A good working knowledge of the muscles of the low back and pelvis is important, and some of the major ones are to be seen in Figures 5.1 and 5.2

TRIGGER POINTS AND PELVIC PAIN

Pelvic pain, interstitial (i.e. unexplained) cystitis and urinary (stress) incontinence

Pelvic pain, and problems of urgency and incontinence, may at times be related to trigger points. However, there may be many other causes of such symptoms, including infection, gynecological disease, pregnancy, weight problems, etc.

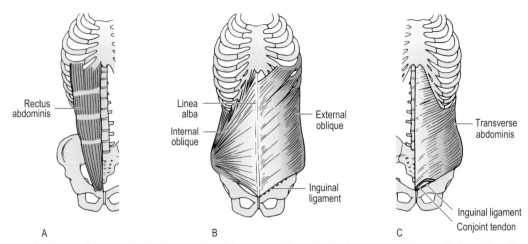

Figure 5.1   (A) Rectus abdominis. (B) Right internal and left external obliques. (C) Left transverse abdominis (Adapted from Braggins 2000 with permission.) (From Chaitow and DeLany 2002.)

As far back as the early 1950s, there were reports that pelvic pain and bladder symptoms, such as cystitis, could be created by trigger points lying in the abdominal muscles (Kelsey 1951).

Travell & Simons (1983), the leading researchers into trigger points, reported that:

> Urinary frequency, urinary urgency and 'kidney' pain may be referred from trigger points in the skin of the lower abdominal muscles. Injection of an old appendectomy scar … has relieved frequency and urgency, and increased the bladder capacity significantly.

More recent research confirms this, and has shown that symptoms such as chronic pelvic pain, and interstitial cystitis, can often be relieved by manual deactivation of trigger points, as well as by injection or acupuncture (Oyama et al 2004, Weiss 2001).

Trigger points and ilio-inguinal nerve entrapment

Understanding how pelvic pain can arise from trigger points (Iyer & Reginald 2000) may be easier if we remind ourselves of the definition:

A trigger point is:

- a hyperirritable focus
- usually found within a taut band of skeletal muscle or in the muscle fascia
- painful on compression
- giving rise to characteristic referred pain, tenderness and autonomic phenomena (Travell & Simons 1992).

Trigger points often appear after tissue injury and are frequently found in the muscles of the anterior abdominal wall and pelvic floor (for example levator ani and coccygeus). Pressure on the trigger points will reproduce the pain symptoms if the triggers are active. Many physicians inject the triggers, or use dry needling or acupuncture to deactivate them, however manual methods are commonly equally effective (Hou et al 2002) and are sometimes more effective (Dardzinski et al 2000).

In some cases, ilio-inguinal nerve entrapment may produce chronic pelvic pain. The nerve may be damaged or entrapped between oblique abdominal muscle fibres, by scar tissue, following surgery. Local anesthetic injections have been shown to relieve this pain in many cases (Hahn 1989).

Trigger points fall into two categories:

1   Close to attachments
2   Close to motor end-points near the bellies of muscles.

This is also true of abdomino-pelvic trigger points, where particular attention should be given to specific junctional tissues, such as:

- the central tendon
- the lateral aspect of the rectal muscle sheaths
- attachment of the recti muscles and external oblique muscles to the ribs
- the xiphisternal ligament, as well as the lower insertions of the internal and external oblique muscles
- intercostal areas from 5th to 12th ribs are equally important
- scars from previous operations.

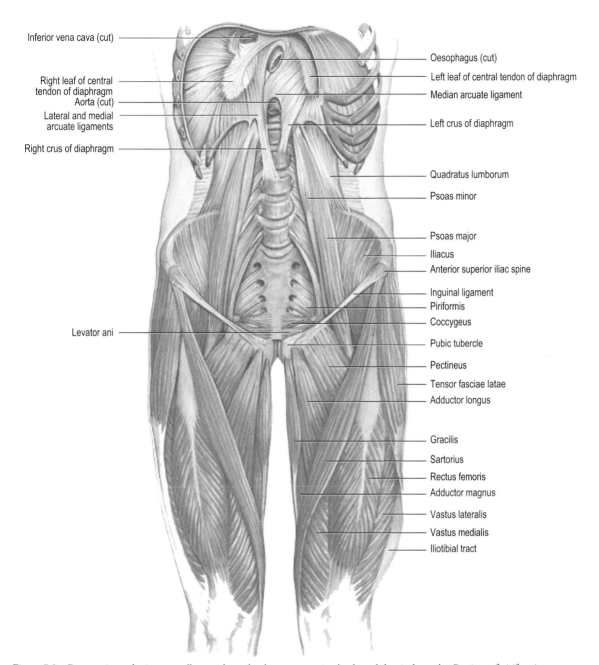

Inferior vena cava (cut)

Right leaf of central
tendon of diaphragm
Aorta (cut)

Lateral and medial
arcuate ligaments

Right crus of diaphragm

Levator ani

Oesophagus (cut)

Left leaf of central tendon of diaphragm

Median arcuate ligament

Left crus of diaphragm

Quadratus lumborum

Psoas minor

Psoas major

Iliacus

Anterior superior iliac spine

Inguinal ligament

Piriformis

Coccygeus

Pubic tubercle

Pectineus

Tensor fasciae latae

Adductor longus

Gracilis

Sartorius

Rectus femoris

Adductor magnus

Vastus lateralis

Vastus medialis

Iliotibial tract

Figure 5.2   Psoas major and minor as well as quadratus lumborum comprise the deep abdominal muscles. Portions of piriformis, coccygeus and levator ani are also shown here. (Reproduced with permission from Gray's Anatomy 1995.) (From Chaitow and DeLany 2002.)

Examples

Pain in the lower abdomen, such as that of dysmenorrhea, may arise from trigger points in the rectus or the lateral abdominal muscles (Figs 5.3, 5.4).

These trigger points can be located during massage, or by carefully searching the tissues where they are housed, as in neuromuscular evaluation (Fig. 5.5).

VISCERAL 'DRAG' AND PELVIC PAIN

Kuchera (1997) points to various ways in which pain and discomfort can arise in the pelvic and abdominal viscera, due to irritation or inflammation.

- A 'vague, gnawing, deep, poorly localized, and mid-abdominal' pain, may derive from irritation of

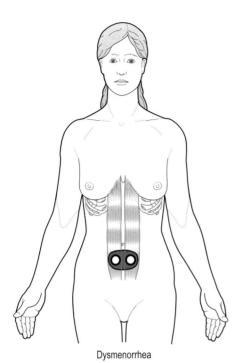

Dysmenorrhea

Figure 5.3   Painful or difficult menstruation (dysmenorrhea) may be due to rectus abdominis trigger points. (Adapted from Simons et al 1999, Figs 49.2A–C.) (From Chaitow and DeLany 2002.)

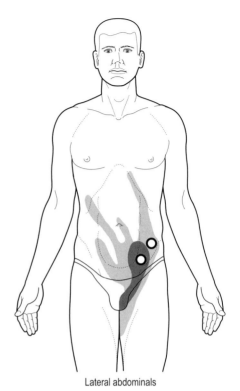

Lateral abdominals

Figure 5.4   Trigger point patterns of lateral abdominal muscles. These patterns may include referrals which affect viscera and provoke viscera-like symptoms, including heartburn, vomiting, belching, diarrhea and testicular pain. (Adapted with permission from Simons et al 1999.) (From Chaitow and DeLany 2002.)

contiguous peritoneal tissues and the abdominal wall
- Abdomino-pelvic pain may be due to reflex pain from different organs, or the spinal cord
- Pain may also derive from a dragging force imposed on the mesentery (the double layer of peritoneal membrane that supports the small intestine) when organs and tissues have sagged (visceroptosis), irritating the peritoneal tissues (Figs 5.6–5.8).

Kuchera (1997) suggests that tenderness and tension in the mesentery can be palpated for tension and treated as follows:

- Place the extended fingers flat over the lateral margin of the ascending or descending colon and moving the viscera towards the midline of the body, monitor for changes in resistance to this movement
- The mesentery of the sigmoid colon is moved towards the umbilicus (Fig. 5.7A)
- Palpate the mesentery, along with the small intestines, by placing the extended fingers carefully into the lower left abdominal quadrant to make indirect contact with as much of the small intestine as possible

- This is moved towards the upper right quadrant of the abdomen (Fig. 5.7B).

To treat restrictions noted in such palpation:

- The patient lies supine, with knees flexed and feet flat on the table
- The therapist's fingers are extended and placed flat over the lateral margin of the mesentery (to be treated) (Fig. 5.8)
- Medial pressure is then applied to the 'restricted' section of bowel, at right angles to its posterior (mesenteric) abdominal wall attachment
- The tension is held as the patient takes a half-breath and holds it. No pain should be produced by this
- After release of the breath the tissues being held should be gently 'turned' clockwise and anticlock-wise, to sense their position of greatest tissue freedom
- The tissues are then held for not less than 90 s, or until a sense of relaxation is noted
- When breathing resumes, after this positional release approach, the tissues should be re-palpated.

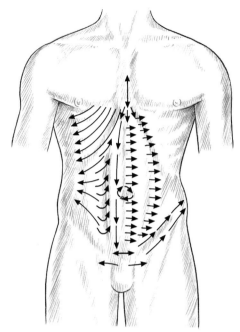

Figure 5.5   Neuromuscular abdominal technique. Suggested lines of application to access primary trigger point attachment sites and interfaces between different muscle groups. (From Chaitow and DeLany 2002.)

Form, force and the self-locking mechanisms of the SIJ

Two mechanisms lock the SI joint physiologically, and these are known as the 'form closure' and 'force closure' mechanisms (Lee 1997) (Fig. 5.9).

- *Form closure* is the state of stability which occurs when the very close fitting joint surfaces of the SI joint approximate, in order to reduce movement opportunities. The efficiency and degree of form closure will vary with size, shape, age, as well as the level of loading involved
- *Force closure* refers to the support offered to the SI joint by the ligaments of the area directly, as well as the various sling systems which involve both muscular and ligamentous structures. It is important to review these extremely important mechanisms by means of which the muscles and ligaments, often acting via connecting fascia, stabilize the SI joints during different phases of activity.

For example:

- During anterior rotation of the ilium or during sacral counter nutation, the SI joint is stabilized by a tightening of the long dorsal sacroiliac ligament

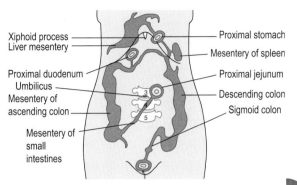

Figure 5.6   Mesenteric attachments as described by Kuchera. From Ward (1997), with permission.

- During sacral nutation, or posterior rotation of the innominate, the SI joint is stabilized by the sacrotuberous and interosseous ligaments.

Muscles that support the SIJ

The inner unit includes:

- the muscles of the pelvic floor (levator ani and coccygeus)
- transversus abdominis
- multifidus
- the diaphragm (Fig. 5.10).

The outer unit comprises four 'systems':

- *Posterior oblique system*: latissimus dorsi, gluteus maximus and the lumbodorsal fascia (which links them). When latissimus and contralateral gluteus maximus contract there is a force closure of the posterior aspect of the SIJ (Fig. 5.11)
- *Deep longitudinal system*: erector spinae, deep laminae of the thoracodorsal fascia, sacrotuberous ligament and biceps femoris. When contraction occurs, biceps femoris influences compression of the SI joint and sacral nutation can be controlled (Fig. 5.12)
- *Anterior oblique system*: external and internal obliques, the contralateral adductors of the thigh and the intervening abdominal fascia. The obliques take part in most upper and lower limb and trunk movements, with transversus abdominis stabilizing. The obliques act almost constantly in unsupported sitting, although crossed-leg posture allows them 'timeout' (Snijders et al 1995) (Fig. 5.13).
- *Lateral system*: gluteus medius and minimus and contralateral adductors of the thigh. It has been suggested that, 'although these muscles are not directly involved in force closure of the SI joint they

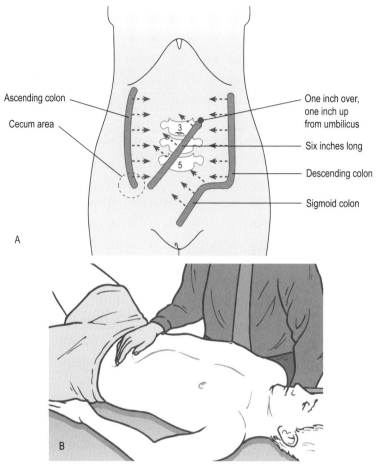

Figure 5.7 (A) Suggested directions of movement in treating intestinal mesentery (after Kuchera). From Ward (1997), with permission. (B) Lifting the small intestine/sigmoid colon to ease mesenteric drag (after Wallace et al). From Ward (1997), with permission.

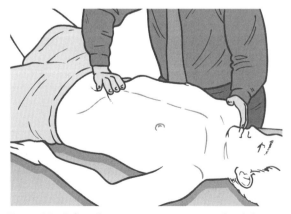

Figure 5.8 Lifting the caecum to ease mesenteric drag (after Wallace et al). From Ward (1997), with permission.

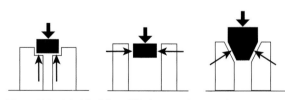

Figure 5.9 Model of the self-locking mechanism: the combination of form closure and force closure establishes stability in the sacroiliac joint (SIJ). (After Vleeming et al 2007.)

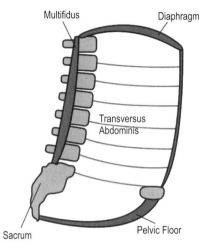

Figure 5.10   The muscles of the inner unit include the multifidus, transversus abdominis, diaphragm and the pelvic floor. (From Lee 2004.)

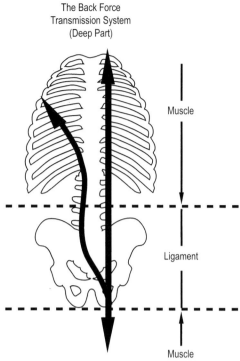

Figure 5.12   The deep longitudinal system of the outer unit consists of erector spinae, the deep laminae of the thoracodorsal fascia, the sacrotuberous ligament and the biceps femoris muscle. (Redrawn from Gracovetsky 1997, from Lee 1999).

Figure 5.11   Schematic dorsal view of the lower back. The right side shows a part of the longitudinal muscle-tendon-fascia sling. Below is the continuation between biceps femoris tendon and sacrotuberous ligament, above a continuation of biceps femoris tendon to the aponeurosis of the erector spinae. To show the right erector spinae, a part of the thoracolumbar fascia ha been removed. The left side shows the sacroiliac joint (O) and the cranial part of the oblique dorsal muscle-fascia-tendon sling: latissimus dorsi muscle and thoracolumbar fascia. In this drawing, the left part of the thoracolumbar fascia is tensed by the left latissimus dorsi and the right gluteus maximus. (Reproduced with permission from Spine). (From Vleeming et al 1997.)

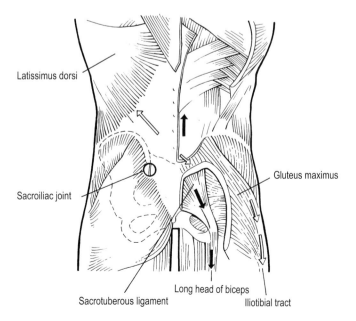

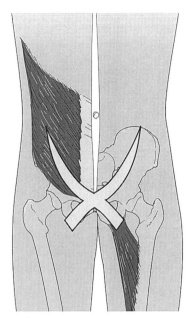

Figure 5.13 The anterior oblique system of the outer unit includes the external and internal oblique, the contralateral adductors of the thigh and the intervening anterior abdominal fascia. (From Lee 2004.)

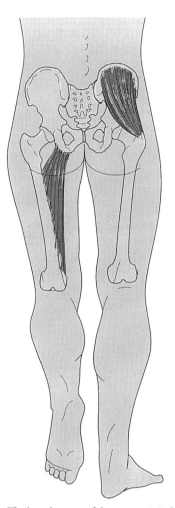

Figure 5.14 The lateral system of the outer unit includes the gluteus medius and minimus and the contralateral adductors of the thigh. (From Lee 1999.)

are significant for the function of the pelvic girdle during standing and walking and are reflexively inhibited when the SI joint is unstable' (Lee 1999) (Fig. 5.14).

Problems

Anything that inhibits or disturbs the main muscles in these processes should be suspect, particularly excessive tone in antagonists to gluteus maximus, minimus and medius, biceps femoris, lumbar erector spinae, multifidus, adductor and abductors of the thigh as well as the oblique abdominals and transversus abdominis.

Inhibition in these muscles may also derive from local or referring trigger points, other forms of local muscular dysfunction (inflammation, fibrosis, etc.) and joint restrictions.

Identification

It is suggested that you examine these important coordinated muscle-ligament-fascia functions, and then carefully read the description (below) of how they function during walking. It is sometimes possible to identify in which part of the gait cycle (for example just before heel-strike, or on toe-off) pain is felt in the

SIJ, so implicating a particular phase of the support system that acts to create supportive compressive force in the SIJ.

- When walking, as the right leg swings forward the right ilium rotates backward in relation to the sacrum (Greenman 1997)
- Simultaneously, the sacrotuberous and interosseous ligamentous tension increases to brace the sacroiliac joint (SIJ) in preparation for heel strike
- Just before heel strike, the ipsilateral hamstrings are activated, thereby tightening the sacrotuberous ligament (into which they merge) to further stabilize the SI joint (Fig. 5.15)

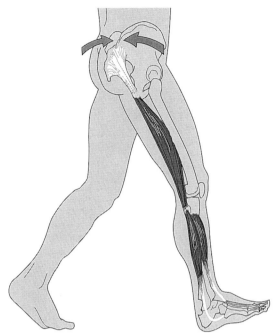

Figure 5.15 At heel strike, posterior rotation of the right innominate increases the tension of the right sacrotuberous ligament. Contraction of the biceps femoris further increases tension in this ligament preparing the sacroiliac joint for impact. (Redrawn from Vleeming et al 1997, from Lee 2004.)

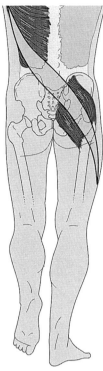

Figure 5.16 During the right single-leg stance phase, contraction of the gluteus maximus and the contralateral latissimus dorsi increases tension through the thoracodorsal fascia and facilitates continued stability of the sacroiliac joint during the weight-bearing phase. (From Lee 2004.)

- As the foot approaches heel-strike, there is a downward movement of the fibula, increasing (via biceps femoris) the tension on the sacrotuberous ligament, while simultaneously tibialis anticus (which attaches to the first metatarsal and medial cuneiform) fires, in order to dorsiflex the foot in preparation for heel strike
- Tibialis anticus links via fascia to peroneus longus (which also attaches to the first metatarsal and medial cuneiform) under the foot; so completing this sling mechanism which both braces the SI joint, and engages the entire lower limb
- Biceps femoris, peroneus longus and tibialis anticus together form the longitudinal muscle-tendon-fascial sling which creates an energy store, to be used during the next part of the gait cycle
- During the latter stage of single support period of the gait cycle, biceps femoris activity eases, as compression of the SI joint reduces and the ipsilateral iliac bone rotates anteriorly
- As the heel strikes, the contralateral arm swings forward – and the gluteus maximus activates to compress and stabilize the SI joint (Fig. 5.16)

- There is a simultaneous coupling of this gluteal force with the contralateral latissimus dorsi by means of thoracolumbar fascia in order to assist in counter-rotation of the trunk on the pelvis
- In this way, an oblique muscle-tendon-fascial sling is created across the torso, providing a mechanism for further energy storage to be utilized in the next phase of the gait cycle
- As the single support phase ends and the double support phase initiates, there is a lessened loading of the SI joints and gluteus maximus reduces its activity, and as the next step starts, the leg swings forward and nutation at the SI joint starts again.

There is ample scope for dysfunction should any of the muscular components become compromised (inhibited, shortened, restricted, etc.). Revisit the assessments in Chapter 4, that allow you to test for weakness and shortness in many of these muscles.

Knowledge of the complex support systems that maintain pelvic and SIJ integrity allows us to use simple tests to evaluate whether pain and dysfunction

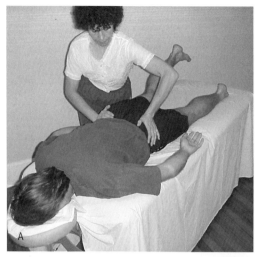

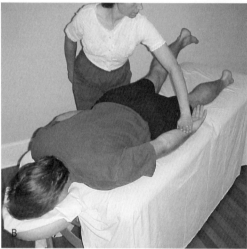

Figure 5.17   Functional test of prone active straight leg raise. (A) With form closure augmented. (B) With force closure augmented. (Adapted from Lee 1999, from Chaitow and DeLany 2002.)

in the SIJ are a result of muscular imbalances ('force') or actual structural problems ('form') in the joint.

Prone active straight leg raising test for the SIJ

- The prone patient is asked to extend the leg at the hip by approximately 10°. Hinging should occur at the hip joint and the pelvis should remain in contact with the table throughout (Fig. 5.17)
- Excessive degrees of pelvic rotation in the transverse plane (anterior pelvic rotation), or marked discomfort when raising the leg, suggests possible SIJ dysfunction
- If *form* features (structural) of the SIJ are at fault, the prone straight leg raise will be more normal when

medial compression of the joint is applied by the therapist, bilaterally applying firm medial pressure towards the SI joints, with hands on the innominates, during the procedure

- *Force* closure may be enhanced during the test if latissimus dorsi can be recruited to increase tension on the thoracolumbar fascia. This is done by the therapist resisting extension of the medially rotated (contralateral) arm before lifting of the leg
- If force closure enhances more normal SIJ function, the prognosis for improvement is good, to be achieved by means of exercise, muscle balancing and reformed use patterns (see Chapters 7,8,9).

Supine active straight leg raising test for the SIJ

- The patient is supine and is asked to raise one leg
- If there is evidence of compensating rotation of the pelvis *towards* the side of the raised leg during performance of the movement, or if there is appreciable discomfort in raising the leg, SIJ dysfunction is strongly suggested
- The same leg should then be raised as the therapist imparts compressive force medially directed across the pelvis, with a hand on the lateral aspect of each innominate, at the level of the ASIS (this assists form closure of the SIJ)
- If *form* closure *as applied by the therapist* enhances the ability to easily raise the leg, this suggests that structural factors within the joint may require external help, such as a supporting belt
- To test *force* closure, the same leg is raised with the patient slightly flexing and rotating the trunk toward the side being tested, against the practitioner's resistance – applied to the contralateral shoulder
- This activates oblique muscular forces and force-closes the SIJ being tested
- If initial leg raising suggests SIJ dysfunction, and this is reduced by means of force-closure, the prognosis is good if the patient engages in appropriate rehabilitation exercise (see Chapters 7,8,9).

Tests for iliosacral and sacroiliac restriction

There are several simple tests that can help to indicate whether pain in the sacroiliac region is being caused by a restriction in that joint.

Further testing can show whether the problem has more to do with iliac, or with sacral, influences (that is, whether this is an iliosacral or a sacroiliac dysfunction).

Why is it important to distinguish between iliosacral and sacroiliac dysfunction?

Imagine a door that is not able to open or close normally due to warping of its structure.

- It is possible that the problem lies with the door itself having warped. Think of the sacrum as the door, which would mean that in this case we would have a sacroiliac joint (SIJ) dysfunction
- Or, it is possible that the frame of the door may have become distorted. Think of the ilia as the frame, which would mean that in this case we would have an iliosacral joint (ISJ) dysfunction
- It is also conceivable that both the door and the frame are contributing to the problem.

There are very simple methods (see Chs 7 and 8), using positional release and/or muscle energy methods, or mobilization with movement (MWM), that can commonly help to normalize such problems, but before using these it is necessary to identify what the problem is.

TESTS

The main tests used to identify ISJ and SIJ problems are the standing and seated flexion tests, with some additional refinements as described below.

A caution is necessary however, as the evidence gained from the standing flexion test, as described below, is invalid if there is concurrent shortness in the hamstrings, since this will effectively give either:

- a false negative result on the side of the shortened hamstrings and/or
- a false positive sign on the side opposite the shortened hamstrings, if there exists unilateral hamstring shortness (due to the restraining influence on the side of hamstring shortness, creating a compensating iliac movement on the other side during flexion); or
- false negative results if there is bilateral hamstring shortness (i.e. there may be iliosacral motion which is masked by the restriction placed on the ilia via hamstring shortness).

Hamstring length testing should therefore be carried out before the standing flexion tests, and if this proves positive, these muscles should be normalized, if appropriate, prior to use of the assessment methods described here.

At the very least, the likelihood of a false positive standing flexion test should be kept in mind if there are hamstring influences of this sort operating.

Similarly, if one or both quadratus lumborum muscles are short, this may distort the accuracy of the test.

Standing flexion (iliosacral) test

- With the patient standing, any apparent inequality of leg length, as suggested by unequal pelvic crest

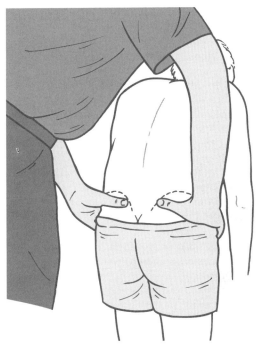

Figure 5.18 Standing flexion test for iliosacral restriction. The dysfunctional side is that on which the thumb moves during flexion. (After Chaitow 2001.)

heights, should be compensated for by insertion of a pad ('shim') under the foot on the short side (Fig. 5.18)
- This helps to avoid errors in judgment as to the end-point positions, for example when assessing the end of range during the standing flexion tests
- The therapist stoops or kneels behind the upright patient, with thumbs placed firmly (a light contact is useless) on the inferior slope of the PSIS
- The patient is asked to go into full flexion while thumb contact is maintained, with the therapist's eyes level with the thumbs
- The patient's knees should remain extended during this bend
- The practitioner observes, *especially near the end of the excursion of the bend*, whether one or other PSIS (thumb) 'travels' more anterosuperiorly than the other (Fig. 5.18).

Interpretation of the standing flexion test
If one thumb moves a greater distance antero-superiorly during flexion it indicates that the ilium is 'fixed' to the sacrum on that side (or that the contra-lateral hamstrings are short, or that the ipsilateral

quadratus lumborum is short; therefore, all these muscles should have been assessed prior to the standing flexion test).

If both hamstrings are excessively short, this may produce a false negative test result, with the flexion potential limited by the muscular shortness, preventing an accurate assessment of iliac movement.

At the end of the flexion excursion, the patient comes back to upright and bends backward, in order to extend the lumbar spine. The PSISs should move equally in an inferior (caudal) direction.

Note: Both the standing flexion test (above) and the 'stork' test (below) are capable of indicating *which side* of the pelvis is most dysfunctional, restricted, hypomobile. They do not however, offer evidence as to *what type* of dysfunction has occurred (i.e. whether it is an anterior or posterior innominate rotation, internal or external innominate flare dysfunction, or something else).

The *nature* of the dysfunction needs to be evaluated by other means, including aspects of supine pelvic assessment as described later.

Standing iliosacral 'stork' or Gillet test

Following the standing flexion test, this test should be performed.

- The therapist places one thumb on the PSIS and the other thumb on the ipsilateral sacral crest, at the same level
- The standing patient flexes knee and hip, and lifts the tested side knee so that he is standing only on one leg
- The normal response would be for the ilium on the tested side (the side where the leg is raised) to rotate posteriorly
- This would bring the thumb on the PSIS caudal and medial (Fig 5.19).

Interpretation of the stork test
Lee (1999) states that this test (if performed on the right), 'examines the ability of the right innominate to posteriorly rotate, the sacrum to right rotate and the L5 vertebrae to right rotate/sideflex'.

If, upon flexion of the knee and hip, the PSIS on that side moves cephalad in relation to the sacrum, this is an indication of both pubic symphysis and iliosacral dysfunction – on that side. This finding can be used to confirm the findings of the standing flexion test (above).

This 'stork' test may also indicate sacroiliac dysfunction on that same side (Petty & Moore 1998). Treatment approaches are discussed in Chapters 7 and 8.

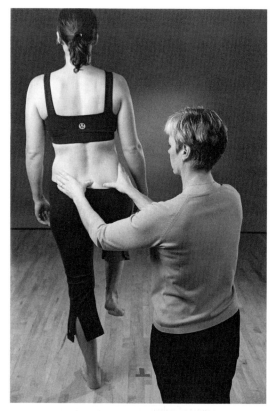

Figure 5.19   Ipsilateral posterior rotation test (Gillet). Note the inferomedial displacement of the PSIS, on the right. (From Chaitow 2006.)

Following the standing flexion test and the stork test, the seated flexion test should be performed.

Positional assessment based on standing flexion test

Once an *iliosacral* dysfunction has been identified by means of the standing flexion test and/or during the stork test, it is necessary to define precisely what type of restriction exists. This depends on observation of landmarks.

Iliosacral dysfunction possibilities include:

- anterior innominate rotation
- posterior innominate rotation
- innominate inflare or outflare
- innominate superior or inferior shear (subluxation).

ROTATIONAL DYSFUNCTIONS

- The patient lies supine, legs flat on the table, and the practitioner approaches the table from the side that allows her dominant eye to be placed directly over the pelvis

- The therapist locates the inferior slopes of the two ASISs (Fig. 5.20) with the thumbs, and views these contacts from directly above the pelvis with the dominant eye over center line (bird's eye view) (Fig. 5.21A)
- The therapist asks her/himself the first question. 'Which ASIS is nearer the head and which nearer the feet?' In other words, is there a possibility that one ilium has rotated posteriorly or the other anteriorly?
- The side of dysfunction will already have been determined by the standing flexion test, and/or the standing hip flexion test (Gillet's stork test). These tests define which observed anterior landmark (left or right) is taken into consideration (the side on which the therapist's thumb moved on flexion)
- If the ASIS appears inferior on the dysfunctional side (compared to the 'normal' side) it is assumed that the ilium has rotated anteriorly on the sacrum on the dysfunctional side (Fig. 5.21B)
- If, however, the ASIS appears superior on the dysfunctional side, then the ilium is assumed to have rotated posteriorly on the sacrum on that side.

See pages 121 and 122 for treatment methods for rotation dysfunction.

FLARE DYSFUNCTIONS

- While observing the ASISs, note is also made as to the positions of these landmarks in relation to the midline of the patient's abdomen by using either the linea alba or the umbilicus as a guide (Fig. 5.21C).
- Is one thumb closer to the umbilicus, or the linea alba, than the other?
- *Remember*: The ASIS on the side on which the PSIS was observed to move superiorly during the flexion test, or during the stork test, is the dysfunctional side
- If the ASIS on that side is closer to the umbilicus it represents an inflare, whereas, if the ASIS is further from the umbilicus, it represents an outflare on that side, and the other side innominate is normal

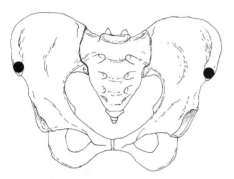

Figure 5.20 Points of palpation of the innominate showing anterior superior iliac spines. (From Chaitow and DeLany 2002.)

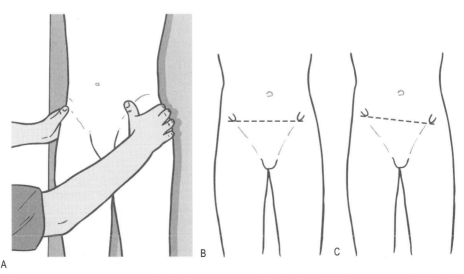

A   B   C

Figure 5.21 (A) Practitioner adopts position so that bird's eye view is possible of palpated ASIS prominences. (B) The ASISs are level, suggesting no rotational dysfunction of the ilia. (C) The right ASIS is higher than the left and if the right thumb had been noted to move during the standing flexion test, this would suggest a posterior right innominate tilt. If the left thumb had moved it would suggest an anterior rotation of the left ilium. (Reproduced with permission from Chaitow 2001.) (After Chaitow and DeLany 2002.)

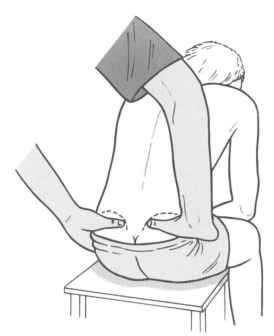

Figure 5.22   Seated flexion test for sacroiliac restriction. The dysfunctional side is the side on which the thumb moves on flexion. (Reproduced with permission from Chaitow 2001.) (After Chaitow and DeLany 2002.)

- Flare dysfunctions are usually treated before rotation dysfunctions.

See page 122 for treatment methods for flare dysfunction.

Note: It is stressed that the MET iliosacral treatment methods as described in Chapter 7 should always be preceded by normalization (as far as possible) of soft tissue influences such as short, tight or weak attaching musculature, including trigger point activity.

Seated flexion (sacroiliac) test

- The patient is seated with feet flat on the floor for support (Fig. 5.22)
- The therapist is behind the patient with thumbs firmly placed on the inferior slopes of the PSISs, fingers placed on the curve of the pelvis, index fingers on the crests, in order to provide stabilizing support for the hands
- The seated flexion test involves observation of thumb movement, if any, during full slowly active flexion.

Interpretation of seated flexion test
Since the weight of the trunk rests on the ischial tuberosities during the test, the ilia cannot easily move, and if one PSIS moves more cephalward during flexion, it suggests a sacroiliac restriction on that side.

A false positive result may be caused by shortness in quadratus lumborum on the side of dysfunction, emphasizing that QL and hamstrings should be evaluated and if necessary treated/stretched before these tests are performed.

See page 121 for treatment method for sacroiliac dysfunction.

SACRAL TENDER POINT ASSESSMENT FOR STRAIN/ COUNTERSTRAIN TREATMENT

Two sets of sacral tender points used in positional release treatment of SI and sacral dysfunction are described below:

1   One set lies on the midline of the sacrum or close to it. These are the so-called 'medial tender points'. They all lie in soft tissues which overlie the bony dorsum of the sacrum so that when digital palpating pressure is applied to them there is a sense of 'hardness' below the point. The characteristic dysfunctions which have been linked to these points are described below as are appropriate treatment approaches. The medial points, as a rule, require a vertical pressure towards the floor, applied in a way which 'tilts' the sacrum sufficiently to relieve the palpated tenderness
2   The other set of sacral points lie over the sacral foramina, and so when pressure is applied to these, there is a sense of 'softness' in the underlying tissues.

In 1989, a series of sacral tender points were identified as being related to low back and pelvic dysfunction. These points were found to be amenable to very simple SCS methods of release (Ramirez 1989).

Subsequently, additional sacral foramen tender points which are believed to relate to sacral torsion dysfunctions were identified (Cislo et al 1991).

LOCATION OF THE SACRAL MEDIAL POINTS

The cephalad two points lie just lateral to the midline, approximately 1.5 cm (3/4 in) medial to the inferior aspect of the PSIS bilaterally, and they are known as PS1 (PS, posterior sacrum).

The two bilateral caudal points (PS5) are located approximately 1 cm (just under 1.2 in) medial, and 1 cm superior to the inferior lateral angles of the sacrum.

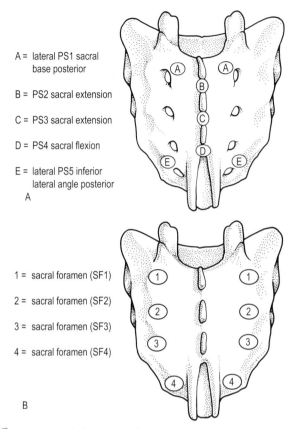

A = lateral PS1 sacral
      base posterior

B = PS2 sacral extension

C = PS3 sacral extension

D = PS4 sacral flexion

E = lateral PS5 inferior
      lateral angle posterior
      A

1 = sacral foramen (SF1)

2 = sacral foramen (SF2)

3 = sacral foramen (SF3)

4 = sacral foramen (SF4)

B

Figure 5.23 (A) Positions of tender points relating to sacral dysfunction (reproduced with permission from Chaitow 1996). (B) Sacral foramen tender points as described in the text (reproduced with permission from Chaitow 1996). (From Chaitow and DeLany 2002.)

The remaining three points are on the midline: one (PS2) lies between the 1st and 2nd spinous tubercles of the sacrum, another lies between the 2nd and 3rd sacral tubercles (PS3), both of which are identified as being involved in sacral extension dysfunctions, and the last point (PS4) lies on the cephalad border of the sacral hiatus – which has been identified as a point relating to sacral flexion dysfunctions.

If you can locate areas of tenderness on the sacrum where the underlying tissues are hard and bony, rather than having a soft feeling just below the surface, you are palpating a sacral medial point. Establish the level of sensitivity when mild pressure is applied and subsequently treat two or three of the most sensitive points (Fig. 5.23).

Treatment of medial sacral tender points:

- Patient prone, press on the sacral tender point being treated

- Pressure is towards the floor, in order to induce rotation/tilting of the sacrum, to ease pain/discomfort by at least 70%
- PS1 points require pressure at the corner of the sacrum opposite the quadrant housing the tender point (i.e. left PS1 requires pressure at right inferior lateral angle)
- PS5 points require pressure near the contralateral sacral base (i.e. right PS5 point requires to the floor pressure at left sacral base, medial to the SI joint)
- Release of PS2 (sacral extension) tender point requires pressure to the floor to the apex of the sacrum in the midline
- Lower PS4 (sacral flexion) tender point requires pressure to the midline of the sacral base
- PS3 (sacral extension) requires the same treatment as for PS2
- Once 'ease' has been achieved, hold the pressure for 60–90 seconds and slowly release.

SACRAL FORAMEN TENDER POINTS

The clinicians who first noted these points reported that a patient with low back pain, with a recurrent sacral torsion, was being treated using SCS methods with poor results. When muscle energy procedures proved inadequate, a detailed survey was made of the region, and an area of sensitivity, which had previously been ignored, was identified in one of the sacral foramina.

If you can locate areas of tenderness on the sacrum where the underlying tissues are 'soft' and spongy, rather than having a feeling of bone just below the surface, you are palpating a foramen point. Establish the level of sensitivity when mild pressure is applied, and subsequently treat two or three of the most sensitive points.

Treatment of sacral foramen tender points:

- The most sensitive of the foramen points are treated. Palpation of the foramina, using skin drag (see Ch. 6 for details) can reveal dysfunction, even if the precise nature of that dysfunction is unclear. If there is obvious skin drag over a foramen, and if compression of that point is painful, sacral torsion exists
- The patient lies prone and you stand on the side of the patient contralateral to the foramen tender point to be treated
- That is, you stand on the right when a left sided foramen point is treated
- Standing on the right, the right leg, flexed at the hip, is abducted to ~30° allowing it to fall slightly over the edge

- While applying pressure to the foramen with your caudal hand, now apply antero-medial pressure to the right ilium, using your right forearm or hand
- Your contact should be ~1 inch (~2.5 cm) lateral to the patient's right PSIS

- Modify angle of pressure on the ilium until the degree of relief of sensitivity at the foramen point is at least 70%
- Hold for 90 seconds before a slow return to neutral.

KEY POINTS

- A great deal of pelvic pain derives from active trigger points
- Pain in the pelvis and low back can be caused by drag on the mesenteric structures, caused by organs that have sagged, or where adhesions exist
- Complex systems of muscular, ligamentous and fascial slings and pulleys support and stabilize the pelvic structures during movement and at rest
- Sacroiliac joint 'force' problems relate to instability caused by muscular imbalances or hypermobility
- Actual structural ('form') features within the joint can also be responsible for SI problems
- Simple tests can establish which is operating in any given situation

- Iliosacral and sacroiliac dysfunction affect precisely the same joint area, but can be primarily caused quite differently, and standing (IS) and seated (SI) flexion tests can help to establish which is which
- Strain/counterstrain methods of treatment utilize 'tender' points located on the sacrum, either on the body surface or over sacral foramina
- Before trying to make sense of the various tests described in this chapter, it is important to normalize as far as possible imbalances (shortness, weakness) in muscles attaching to the pelvis, particularly hamstrings, quadratus lumborum, tensor fascia lata and piriformis.

References

Braggins S 2000 Back care: a clinical approach. Churchill Livingstone, Edinburgh

Chaitow L 2001 Muscle energy techniques, 2nd edn. Churchill Livingstone, Edinburgh

Chaitow L 2003 Modern neuromuscular techniques, 2nd edn. Churchill Livingstone, Edinburgh

Chaitow L 2006 Muscle energy techniques, 3rd edn. Churchill Livingstone, Edinburgh

Chaitow L, DeLany J 2002 Clinical applications of neuromuscular technique, Volume 2. Churchill Livingstone, Edinburgh

Cislo S, Ramirez M, Schwartz H 1991 Low back pain: treatment of forward and backward sacral torsion using counterstrain technique. Journal of the American Osteopathic Association 91(3):255–259

Dardzinski J, Ostrov B, Hamann L 2000. Myofascial pain unresponsive to standard treatment. Successful use of a strain and counterstrain technique with physical therapy. Journal of Clinical Rheumatology 6(4):169–174

Gracovetsky S 1997 Linking the spinal engine with the legs: a theory of human gait. In: Vleeming A, Mooney V, Dorman T, Snijders C, Stoeckart R (eds) Movement, stability and low back pain. Churchill Livingstone, Edinburgh

Gray's Anatomy 1995 (38th edn.) Churchill Livingstone, Edinburgh

Greenman P 1997 Clinical aspects of the SIJ in walking. In: Vleeming A, Mooney V, Dorman T, Snijders C, Stoeckart R (eds) Movement, stability and low back pain. Churchill Livingstone, Edinburgh

Hahn L 1989 Clinical findings and results of operative treatment in ilio-inguinal nerve entrapment. British Journal of Obstetrics and Gynaecology (96):1080–1083

Hou C-R, Tsai L-C, Cheng K-F et al 2002 Immediate effects of various physical therapeutic modalities on cervical myofascial pain and trigger-point sensitivity. Archives of Physical Medicine and Rehabilitation 83:1406–1414

Iyer L, Reginald P 2000 Management of chronic pelvic pain. Current Obstetrics & Gynaecology 10:208–213

Kelsey M 1951 Diagnosis of upper abdominal pain. Texas State Journal of Medicine 47:82–86

Kuchera W 1997 Lumbar and abdominal region. In: Ward R (ed.) Foundations of osteopathic medicine. Williams and Wilkins, Baltimore, p 581–599

Lee D 1997 Treatment of pelvic instability. In: Vleeming A, Mooney V, Dorman T, Snijders C, Stoeckart R (eds) Movement, stability and low back pain. Churchill Livingstone, Edinburgh

Lee D 1999 The pelvic girdle, 2nd edn. Churchill Livingstone, Edinburgh

Lee D 2004 The pelvic girdle, 3rd edn. Churchill Livingstone, Edinburgh

Oyama I, Rejba A, Lukban J et al 2004 Modified Thiele massage as therapeutic intervention for female patients with interstitial cystitis and high-tone pelvic floor dysfunction. Urology 64(5):862–886

Petty N, Moore A 1998 Neuromusculoskeletal examination and assessment. Churchill Livingstone, Edinburgh

Ramirez M 1989 Low back pain – diagnosis by six newly discovered sacral tender points and treatment with counterstrain technique. Journal of the American Osteopathic Association 89(7):905–913

Simons D, Travell J, Simons L 1999 Myofascial pain and dysfunction: the trigger point manual, vol 1, upper half of body, 2nd edn. Williams and Wilkins, Baltimore

Snijders C, Bakker M, Vleeming A, et al 1995 Oblique abdominal muscle activity in standing and sitting on hard and soft seats. Clinical Biomechanics 10(2):73–78

Travell J, Simons D 1983 Myofascial pain and dysfunction: The trigger point manual, Vol. 1, Upper body, 1st edn. Williams & Wilkins, Baltimore, p 671

Travell J G, Simons D G 1992 Myofascial pain and dysfunction: The trigger point manual, Vol. 2. Williams & Wilkins, Baltimore

Vleeming A, Mooney V, Dorman T, Snijders C, Stoeckart R (eds) 1997 Movement, stability and low back pain: the essential role of the pelvis. Churchill Livingstone, Edinburgh

Vleeming R, Mooney V, Stoeckart R 2007 Movement, stability and lumbopelvic pain, 2nd edn. Churchill Livingstone, Edinburgh

Vleeming A, Snijders C J, Stoeckart R, Mens J M A 1997 The role of the sacroiliac joints in coupling between spine, pelvis, legs and arms. In: Vleeming A, Mooney V, Dorman T, Snijders C, Stoeckart R (eds) Movement, stability and low back pain. Churchill Livingstone, Edinburgh

Ward R (ed) 1997 Foundations for osteopathic medicine. Williams and Wilkins, Baltimore

Weiss J 2001 Pelvic floor myofascial trigger points: manual therapy for interstitial cystitis and the urgency-frequency syndrome. Journal of Urology 166:2226–2231

Chapter 6

Modalities working with massage

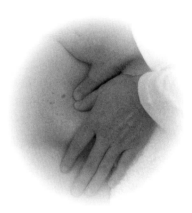

In this chapter, a number of modalities that integrate well with massage therapy will be discussed, together with some practical examples and skill enhancement exercises.

The methods that will be outlined in this way include:

1 Palpation skills
2 Neuromuscular technique
3 Muscle energy technique
4 Positional release technique
5 Spray-and-stretch chilling methods
6 Integrated neuromuscular inhibition (for trigger point deactivation)
7 Rehabilitation exercise methods
8 Massage evidence.

In Chapter 7 and Chapter 8, these methods will be expanded on and described in the context of massage sessions.

PALPATION SKILLS

The ability of a therapist to regularly and accurately locate and identify somatic landmarks, and changes in function, lies at the heart of palpation skills.

Greenman (1996) has summarized the five objectives of palpation. You, the therapist, should be able to:

- detect abnormal tissue texture
- evaluate symmetry in the position of structures, both physically and visually
- detect and assess variations in range and quality of movement during the range, as well as the quality of the end of the range of any movement ('end feel')
- sense the position in space of yourself and the person being palpated
- detect and evaluate changes, whether these are improving or worsening as time passes.

Perspectives

Stone (1999) describes palpation as the 'fifth dimension':

> Palpation allows us to interpret tissue function ... a muscle feels completely different from a ligament, a bone and an organ, for example. There is a 'normal' feel to healthy tissues that is different for each tissue. This has to be learned through repeated exploration of 'normal' as the [therapist] builds his/her own vocabulary of what 'normal' is. Once someone is trained to use palpation efficiently, then finer and finer differences between tissues can be felt ... one must be able to differentiate when something has changed from being 'normal' to being 'too normal'.

Maitland (2001) has commented:

> In the vertebral column, it is palpation that is the most important and the most difficult skill to learn. To achieve this skill, it is necessary to be able to feel, by palpation, the difference in the spinal segments – normal to abnormal, old or new, hypomobile or hypermobile – and then to be able to relate the response, site, depth and relevance to a patient's symptoms (structure, source and causes). This requires an honest, self-critical attitude, and also applies to the testing of functional movements and combined physiological test movements.

Kappler (1997) explains:

> The art of palpation requires discipline, time, patience and practice. To be most effective and productive, palpatory findings must be correlated with a knowledge of functional anatomy, physiology and pathophysiology ... Palpation with fingers and hands provides sensory information that the brain interprets as: temperature, texture, surface humidity, elasticity, turgor, tissue tension, thickness, shape, irritability, motion. To accomplish this task, it is necessary to teach the fingers to feel, think, see, and know. One feels through the palpating fingers on the patient; one sees the structures under the palpating fingers through a visual image based on knowledge of anatomy; one thinks what is normal and abnormal, and one knows with confidence acquired with practice that what is felt is real and accurate.

ARTT

In osteopathic medicine the locality of a dysfunctional musculoskeletal area is noted as having a number of common characteristics, summarized by the acronym ARTT (**A**symmetry, **R**ange of motion, **T**issue texture changes, **T**issue tenderness (sometimes rearranged as TART) (Gibbons & Tehan 2001). These characteristics describe the basis of osteopathic palpation, when assessing for somatic dysfunction:

A relates to Asymmetry
This evaluates functional or structural differences when comparing one side of the body with the other

R relates to Range of motion
Alteration in range of motion can apply to a single joint, several joints, or a muscle. The abnormality may be either restricted or increased mobility, and includes assessment of range as well as *quality* of movement and *'end feel'*.

T relates to Tissue texture changes
The identification of tissue texture change is important in the diagnosis of somatic dysfunction. Palpable changes may be noted in superficial, intermediate and deep tissues. It is important for a therapist to be able to distinguish 'normal' from 'abnormal', even if the nature of the change, or the cause(s), remain unclear.

T relates to Tissue tenderness
Unusual levels of tissue tenderness may be evident. Pain provocation and reproduction of familiar symptoms are often used to localize somatic dysfunction such as trigger points.

Skin assessment and palpation

Changes in the skin, above areas of dysfunction ('hyperalgesic skin zones'), where the tissues may be inflamed, or where there is increased hypertonicity or spasm, or where there have been trigger point changes, are easily palpated (Bischof & Elmiger 1960, Reed & Held 1988).

- The skin adheres to the underlying fascia more efficiently, and is therefore more resistant to movements such as sliding (on underlying fascia), lifting, or rolling
- The skin displays increased sympathetic activity, resulting in increased hydrosis (sweat). This sudomotor activity brings about a noticeable resistance during light stroking with (say) a finger. This resistance is known in clinical shorthand as 'skin drag'
- The skin appears to be more 'compacted', resisting effective separation, stretching, lifting methods
- The skin displays altered thermal qualities, allowing for some discrimination between such areas and normal surrounding tissue.

Tests

The three methods described below do not need to be used during the same treatment session, although they can be. The methods described can support or replace each other, with some therapists having a preference for one or the other.

Note: It is easier to displace skin against underlying tissue in slim individuals, with little fatty tissue. Obese individuals have a higher fat and water content subcutaneously, making displacement more difficult.

Skin on fascia displacement (Fig. 6.1)
- The patient lies prone with the therapist standing to the side, at hip level, contacting the patient with both hands (or the pads of several fingers of each hand) flat against the skin bilaterally, at sacral level
- Only enough pressure should be used to produce adherence between the fingertips and the skin (no lubricant should be used at this stage)
- The skin and subcutaneous tissues should be lightly moved ('slid') towards the head, simultaneously on each side, against the fascia by small pushing movements of the hands, assessing for the elastic barrier
- It is important that areas on both left and right of the spine are examined at the same time
- The two sides should be compared for symmetry of range of movement of the skin and subcutaneous tissue, to the elastic barrier
- The pattern of testing should be performed from inferior to superior

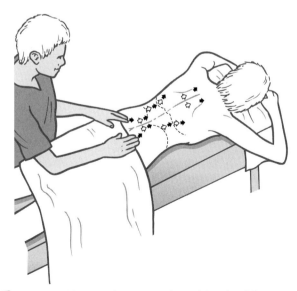

Figure 6.1   Testing and comparing skin and fascial mobility as bilateral areas are 'pushed' to their elastic barriers.

- The degree of displacement possible should be symmetrical, if the deeper tissues are normal
- It should be possible to identify local areas where the skin adherence to underlying connective tissue reveals restriction, compared with the opposite side
- This is likely to be an area where the muscles beneath the skin being tested house active myofascial trigger points (TrPs), or tissue that is dysfunctional in some other way, or hypertonic.

It is often possible to visualize these reflex areas as they may be characterized by being retracted or elevated, most commonly close to the lower thoracic border of the scapula and over the pelvic and gluteal areas.

Skin stretching assessment (Fig. 6.2)
Note: At first, this method should be practiced slowly. Eventually, it should be possible to move fairly rapidly over an area that is being searched for evidence of reflex activity (or acupuncture points). Choose an area to be assessed, where you identified abnormal degrees of skin on fascia adherence.

- To examine the back region, the patient should be lying prone
- Place your two index fingers next to each other, on the skin, side by side or pointing towards each other, with no pressure at all onto the skin, just a contact touch
- Lightly and slowly separate your fingers, feeling the skin stretch to its 'easy' limit, to the barrier where resistance is first noted
- It should be possible – in normal tissue – to 'spring' the skin further apart, to its elastic limit, from that barrier
- Release this stretch and move both fingers 1.2 cm (1/2 in) to one side, or below, or above, the first test site, and repeat the assessment again, using the same direction of pull as you separate the fingers. Add a spring assessment once the barrier is reached
- Perform exactly the same sequence over and over again, until the entire area of tissue has been searched, ensuring that the rhythm you use is neither too slow nor too rapid. Ideally, one stretch per second should be performed
- When the segment of skin being stretched is not as elastic as it was on the previous stretch a potential dysfunctional area will have been identified
- This should be marked with a skin pencil for future attention
- Light digital pressure to the center of that small zone may identify a sensitive contracture which, on sustained pressure, may radiate or refer sensations to a distant site

Figure 6.2 (A,B) Hyperalgesic skin zones that lie above reflexive dysfunction (e.g. trigger points) are identified by means of the sequential stretching to their elastic barrier of local areas of skin. A series of such stretches indicates precisely those areas where elasticity is reduced in comparison to surrounding tissues. These are then tested for sensitivity and potential to cause referred pain by the application of ischemic compression (inhibition). (From Chaitow 2003a.)

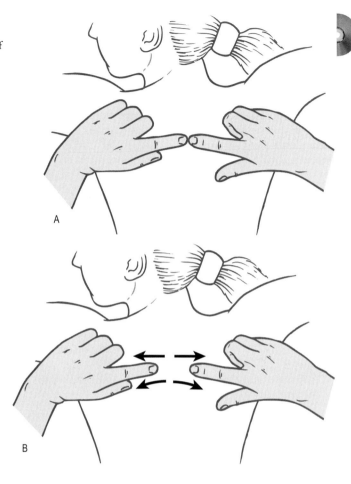

- If such sensations are familiar to the patient, the point being pressed is an active trigger point.

Drag palpation assessment (Fig. 6.3)

Sweat glands, controlled by the sympathetic nervous system, empty directly on the skin, creating increased hydrosis (sweat) presence, changing the behavior (e.g. elasticity) and 'feel' of the skin (Adams et al 1982).

Lewit (1999) suggests that reflex activity should be easily identified by assessing the degree of elasticity in the overlying skin, and comparing it with surrounding tissue.

The change in elasticity occurs at the same time as increased sweat activity. Before the days of electrical detection of acupuncture points, skilled acupuncturists could quickly identify 'active' points by palpation using this knowledge. It is also the reason why measuring the electrical resistance of the skin can now find acupuncture points even more rapidly. Because the skin is moist, it conducts electricity more efficiently than when it is dry.

Method

- Using an extremely light touch ('skin on skin'), without any pressure, a finger or the thumb is stroked across the skin overlaying areas suspected of housing dysfunctional changes (such as TrPs)
- The areas chosen are commonly those where skin-on-fascia movement (see previous test) was reduced, compared with surrounding skin
- When the stroking finger passes over areas where a sense of hesitation, or 'drag,' is noted, an area of increased hydrosis/sweat/sympathetic activity will have been identified
- A degree of searching pressure, into such tissues, precisely under the area of drag, may locate a taut band of tissue, and when this is compressed a painful response is common

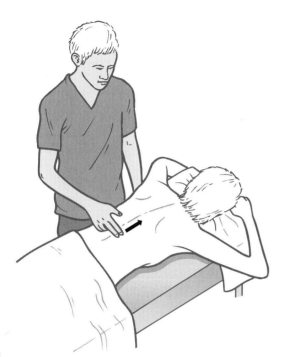

Figure 6.3 Assessing variations in skin friction (drag, resistance).

- If pressure is maintained for 2–3 s a radiating or referred sensation (possibly pain) may be reported
- If this sensation replicates symptoms previously noted by the patient, the point located is an active TrP.

Therapeutic use of skin changes

Releasing skin changes by stretching
- Return to a hyperalgesic skin zone identified by one of the methods described above. Gently stretch the skin to its elastic barrier and hold it at the elastic barrier for 10–15 s, without force
- You should feel the skin tightness gradually release so that, as you hold the elastic barrier, your fingers separate
- If you now hold the skin in its new stretched position, at its new barrier of resistance, for a few seconds longer, it should release a little more
- This is, in effect, a mini-myofascial release process
- The tissues beneath the 'released' skin will be more pliable and have improved circulation. You will have started the process of normalization
- Larger areas, superficial to tense muscles in the low back, for example, can be treated in much the same way as the small skin areas described above (Fig. 6.4)

Box 6.1   Summary of skin palpation methods

- Movement of skin on fascia: resistance indicates general locality of reflexogenic activity, a 'hyperalgesic skin zone' such as a trigger point
- Local loss of skin elasticity: refines definition of the location
- Light stroke, seeking 'drag' sensation (increased hydrosis), offers pinpoint accuracy of location.

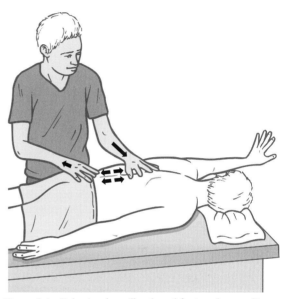

Figure 6.4 Releasing the axillary lateral fascia and pectoralis fibers (abdominal attachments). (Redrawn from Lewit 1996).

- Using a firm contact, place the full length of the sides of both hands, from the little fingers to the wrist, onto an area of skin on the low back (as an example) overlying tense muscles
- Separate the hands slowly, stretching the skin with which they are in contact, until an elastic barrier is reached
- After 15 s or so, there should be a sense of lengthening as the superficial tissues release
- If you then palpate the underlying muscles and areas of local tension you should be able to confirm that there has been a change for the better.

Adding an isometric contraction
If you had asked the patient to lightly contract the muscles under your hands for 5–7 s before starting the myofascial release, the tissues would probably have

responded more rapidly and effectively. You would have been using muscle energy technique (MET), described further later in the chapter.

Positional release method
- Locate an area of skin that tested as 'tight' when you evaluated it, using one of the assessment methods described earlier
- Place two or three finger pads onto the skin and slide the skin superiorly and then inferiorly on the underlying fascia
- In which direction did the skin slide most easily and furthest?
- Slide the skin in *that* direction and now, while holding it there, test the preference of the skin to slide medially and laterally
- Which of these is the 'easiest' direction?
- Slide the tissue towards this second position of ease
- Now introduce a gentle clockwise and anticlockwise twist to these tissues
- Which way does the skin feel most comfortable as it rotates?
- Take it in *that* direction, so that you are now holding the skin in three 'stacked' positions of ease (Fig. 6.5)
- Hold this for not less than 20 s
- Release the skin and retest; it should now display a far more symmetrical preference in all the directions which were previously 'tight'
- The underlying tissues should palpate as softer and less tense.

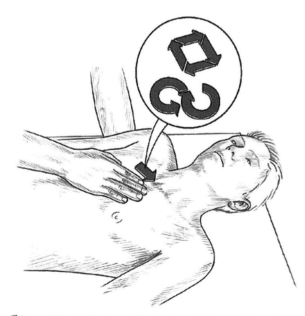

Figure 6.5 Achieving positional release of tissues – skin and fascia – by holding them in their preferred 'ease' directions. From Chaitow (2002), with permission.

Findings

1 You have now established that holding skin at its barrier (unforced) changes its function, as the skin releases
2 You will also have discovered that by adding a very light isometric contraction before the stretch it is even more effective
3 This last example will have shown you that moving tissues away from the barrier into ease (positional release technique) can also achieve a release. This last approach is more suitable for very painful, acute, situations.

NEUROMUSCULAR TECHNIQUE ASSESSMENT AND TREATMENT METHODS

The palpating hand(s) needs to uncover the locality, nature, degree and if possible the age of dysfunctional soft-tissue changes that may have taken place, and as we palpate we need to ask:

- Is this palpable change acute or chronic (or, as is often the case, an acute phase of a chronic condition)?
- If acute, is there any inflammation associated with the changes?
- How do these palpable soft tissue changes relate to the patient's symptom pattern?
- Are these palpable changes part of a pattern of stress-induced change that can be mapped and understood?
- Are these soft tissue changes painful and if so, what is the nature of that pain (constant, intermittent, sharp, dull, etc.)?
- Are these palpable changes active reflexively, and if so, are active or latent trigger points involved (that is, do they refer symptoms elsewhere, and if so does the patient recognize the pain as part of their symptom picture)?
- Are these changes present in a postural or phasic muscle group (see Ch. 1)?
- Are these palpable changes the result of joint restriction ('blockage', subluxation, lesion) or are they contributing to such dysfunction?

In other words, we need to ask ourselves 'What am I feeling, and what does it mean?'

Neuromuscular technique (NMT) evolved in Europe in the 1930s as a blend of traditional Ayurvedic (Indian) massage techniques and soft-tissue methods derived from other sources. Stanley Lief DC and his cousin Boris Chaitow ND DO developed the techniques now known as NMT into an excellent and economical diagnostic (and therapeutic) tool (Chaitow 2003a, Youngs 1962). There is also an American version of NMT that emerged from the work of chiropractor Raymond Nimmo (Cohen & Gibbons 1998).

Trigger points

The major sites of trigger points are often close to the origins and insertions of muscles and this is where NMT probes for information more effectively than most other systems.

Lief (Chaitow 2003a) advocated that the same sequence of contacts be followed at each treatment session, whether assessing or treating, the difference between these modes (assessment and treatment) being merely one of repetition of the strokes, with a degree of added pressure when treating.

Lief's recommendation did not, however, mean that the same treatment was given each time, for the essence of NMT is that the pressure applied, both in diagnosis and in therapy, is variable, and that this variability is determined by the changes located in the tissues themselves.

Basics of NMT

- A light lubricant is always used in NMT, to avoid skin drag
- The main contact is made with the tip of the thumb(s), more precisely the medial aspect of the tip
- In some regions the tip of the index or middle finger is used instead as this allows easier insertion between the ribs for assessment (or treatment) of, for example, intercostal musculature.

Neuromuscular thumb technique
The therapist uses the medial tip (ideally) of the thumb to sequentially 'meet and match' tissue density/ tension and to insinuate the digit through the tissues seeking local dysfunction (Fig. 6.6).

Neuromuscular finger technique
The therapist utilizes the index or middle finger, supported by a neighboring digit (or two), to palpate and assess the tissues between the ribs for local dysfunction. This contact is used instead of the thumb if it is unable to maintain the required pressure (Fig. 6.7).

Posture and positioning

- The therapist's posture and positioning are particularly important when applying NMT, as the correct application of forces dramatically reduces the energy expended and the time taken to perform the assessment/treatment
- The examination table should be at a height which allows the therapist to stand erect, legs separated

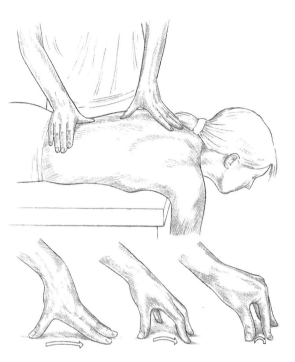

Figure 6.6 Neuromuscular (NMT) thumb technique. (From Chaitow 2003a.)

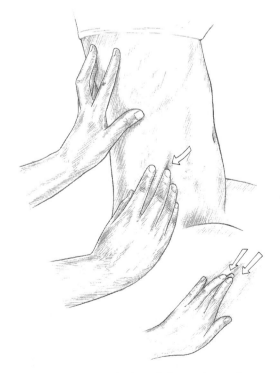

Figure 6.7 Neuromuscular (NMT) finger technique. (From Chaitow 2003a.)

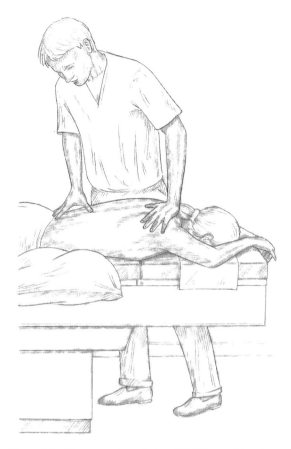

Figure 6.8 Neuromuscular technique (NMT): practitioner's posture should ensure a straight treating arm for ease of transmission of body weight, as well as leg positions that allow for the easy transfer of weight and center of gravity. These postures assist in reducing energy expenditure and ease spinal stress. (From Chaitow 2003a.)

for ease of weight transference, with the assessing arm straight at the elbow. This allows the therapist's body weight to be transferred down the extended arm through the thumb, imparting any degree of force required, from extremely light to quite substantial, simply by leaning on the arm (Fig. 6.8).

The NMT thumb stroke

- It is important that the fingers of the assessing/treating hand act as a fulcrum and that they lie at the front of the contact, allowing the stroke made by the thumb to run across the palm of the hand, towards the ring or small finger as the stroke progresses (Fig. 6.6)
- The finger/fulcrum remains stationary as the thumb draws intelligently towards it, across the

palm. This is quite different from a usual massage stroke, in which the whole hand moves. Here the hand is stationary and only the thumb moves

- Each stroke, whether it be diagnostic or therapeutic, extends for approximately 4–5 cm before the thumb ceases its motion, at which time the fulcrum/fingers can be moved further ahead in the direction the thumb needs to travel
- The thumb stroke then continues, feeling and searching through the tissues
- Another vital ingredient, indeed the very essence of the thumb contact, is its application of variable pressure (diagnostic pressure is in ounces or grams initially) which allows it to 'insinuate' and tease its way through whatever fibrous, indurated or contracted structures it meets
- A degree of vibrational contact, as well as the variable pressure, allows the stroke and the contact to have an 'intelligent' feel and seldom risk traumatizing or bruising tissues, even when heavy pressure is used.

Patterns: NMT maps

The pattern of strokes which Lief and Chaitow evolved allows maximum access to potential dysfunction in the shortest time and with least demand for altered position and wasted effort.

These strokes are applied to the low back area with the suggested therapist foot positions shown in (Figs 6.9A,B, 6.10A,B).

Application of NMT

- Diagnostic assessment involves one superficial and one moderately deep contact only
- If treatment is decided on at that time then several more strokes, applied from varying angles, would be used to relax the structures, to stretch them, to inhibit contraction, or to deal with trigger points discovered during the examination phase
- When assessing (or treating) joint dysfunction, it is suggested that all the muscles associated with a joint receive NMT attention to origins and insertions, and that the bellies of the muscles be searched for evidence of trigger points and other dysfunctions (fibrosis, contractions, etc.)
- A full spinal NMT assessment can be accomplished in approximately 15 min with ease, once the method is mastered
- However, a diagnostic evaluation of a localized region, e.g. covering the area above and below the crest of the pelvis, accompanied by other diagnostic and assessment modalities and methods, may be all that is necessary

Figure 6.9 (A,B) Sixth positions of suggested sequence of applications of neuromuscular technique (NMT). (From Chaitow 2003a.)

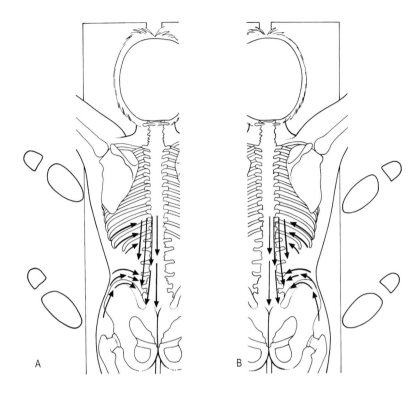

Figure 6.10 (A,B) Seventh positions of suggested sequence of applications of neuromuscular technique (NMT). (From Chaitow 2003a.)

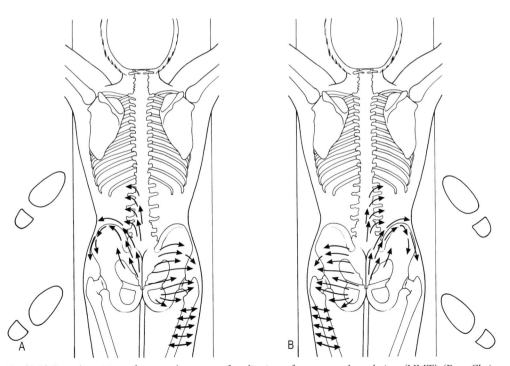

- With effective use of NMT, not only would localized, discrete 'points' be discovered, but also patterns of stress bands, altered soft tissue mechanics, contractions and shortenings.

NMT exercises: finger and thumb strokes

- Apply a light lubricant, position yourself (Figs 6.8, 6.9), and place your treating hand with your fingers acting as a fulcrum, and the thumb (medial tip) feeling through the tissues, slowly and with variable pressure
- Practice this, in no particular sequence of strokes, until the mechanics of the body-arm-hand-thumb positions are comfortable and require no thought
- Pay attention to varying the pressure, to *meeting and matching tension in the tissues*, and to using body weight, transferred through a straight arm, to increase pressure when needed
- Also practice the use of the finger stroke, especially on curved areas, by drawing the slightly hooked and supported (by one of its neighboring digits) finger towards yourself, in a slow, deliberate, searching manner
- Follow the strokes precisely as illustrated in Figures 6.9, 6.10, although the direction of strokes need not follow arrow directions
- The objective is to obtain information, without causing excessive discomfort to the patient, and without stressing your palpating hands
- In its treatment mode NMT involves using greater pressure in order to modify dysfunctional tissues, but in these sequences you can, if you wish, focus on 'information gathering' only, not treating
- In time, with practice, treatment and assessment meld seamlessly together, with one feeding the other
- Chart any findings you make: tender areas, stress bands, contracted fibers, edematous areas, nodular structures, hypertonic regions, trigger points and so on
- If trigger points are located, note their target area as well.

MUSCLE ENERGY TECHNIQUE

Are the tissues you are assessing tense or relaxed? Can your palpating hands identify 'ease' and 'bind'?

The tissues provide the palpating hands or fingers with a sense of these states, and there can never be enough focus on these two characteristics, which allow the tissues to speak as to their current degree of activity, comfort or distress. Ward (1997) states that 'Tightness suggests tethering, while looseness suggests joint and/or soft tissue laxity, with or without neural inhibition'.

Most problems of the musculoskeletal system involve, as part of their etiology, dysfunction related to muscle shortening (Janda 1978, Liebenson 1996).

Where weakness (lack of tone) is apparently a major element, it will often be found that antagonists are shortened, reciprocally inhibiting their tone, and that prior to any effort to strengthen weak muscles, hypertonic antagonists should be dealt with by appropriate means (such as MET, see below), after which spontaneous toning occurs in the previously hypotonic or relatively weak muscles.

If tone remains reduced, then, and only then, should there be specific focus on toning weak muscles (Lewit 1999).

Which method should you choose, PIR or RI?

The presence of pain is frequently the deciding factor in choosing one or other of the methods described (PIR or RI) – contracting the agonist or the antagonist.

When using PIR, the very muscles which have shortened are being contracted.

If the condition of the area is one in which there is a good deal of pain, where any contraction could well trigger more pain, it might be best to avoid using these

---

Box 6.2   Muscle energy technique summary

- By lightly contracting a short, tight muscle isometrically (the agonist) for approximately 7 s, an effect known as post-isometric relaxation (PIR) is produced. This offers an opportunity to stretch the previously shortened muscle(s) more effectively
- By lightly contracting the antagonists to tight/short muscles, an effect known as reciprocal inhibition (RI) is produced in the affected muscle(s), and this also offers an opportunity to stretch the previously shortened muscle(s) more effectively
- A process known as 'increased tolerance to stretch' (ITS) is produced by isometric contractions (i.e. MET) of the agonist(s), the muscle(s) needing lengthening, or their antagonists. This ITS effect means that you can more easily (because the muscle will be more relaxed) introduce greater force into a stretch than you could have done without the isometric contraction, because a neurological change will have taken place, reducing the sensitivity of the patient (Ballantyne et al 2003, Rowlands et al 2003).

The aim is to contract the shortened muscles, or their antagonists, in order to achieve the release of tone and to then be able, with greater ease, to stretch the muscle(s).

muscles, and choose the antagonists instead. Use of the antagonists (inducing RI) might therefore be your first choice for MET when the shortened muscles are very sensitive.

Later, when pain has been reduced by means of MET (or other) methods, PIR techniques (which use isometric contraction of the already shortened muscles rather than the antagonists used in RI methods) could be tried.

To a large extent, just how acute or chronic a condition is helps to decide the method best suited to treating it.

Both methods (PIR and RI) will produce a degree of increased tolerance to stretch.

The essential variables of MET

- The amount of effort used in the contraction effort
- Other major variables that are controllable are, how long the contraction is allowed to continue, and how often it is repeated
- The degree of effort in isometric contractions should always be much less than the full force available from the muscles involved
- The initial contraction should involve the use of a quarter or less of the strength available
- This is never an exact measurement, but indicates that we do not ever want a wrestling match to develop between the contracting area controlled by the patient, and the counterforce offered by you
- After the initial slowly commenced contraction, subsequent contractions may involve an increase in effort, but should never reach more than half of the full strength of that muscle
- We want above all to achieve a controlled degree of effort at all times, and this calls for the use of only part of the available strength in a muscle or muscle group
- The timing of isometric contractions is usually such as to allow around 7 s for the contraction, from beginning to end
- It is important to remember that the start and the end of contraction should always be slow. There should never be a rapid beginning or end to the contraction
- Always attempt a smooth build-up of power in the muscle(s) and a slow switch-off of the contraction at the end. This will prevent injury or strain, and allows for the best possible results
- Contractions should always commence with the shortened muscle held close to its end of range, but, for comfort, never while it is already at stretch

- After the isometric contraction, assisted by the patient, you should move the muscle past its previous barrier, into a slight stretch, and this should be held for not less than 30 s to achieve slow lengthening
- No pain should be caused
- If there is pain you may have taken the muscle into an excessive degree of stretch
- Each stretch should be repeated twice.

MET exercises

Before starting this exercise (Greenman 1996, Goodridge & Kuchera 1997), ensure that the patient lies supine, so that the non-tested leg is abducted slightly, with the heel over the end of the table (Fig. 6.11A,B).

Post isometric relaxation (PIR)
- The leg to be tested should be close to the edge of the table
- Ensure that the tested leg is in the anatomically correct position, knee in full extension and with no external rotation of the leg, which would negate the test
- Holding the patient's foot/ankle, you slowly ease the straight leg into abduction
- Stop the abduction when you sense that a barrier of resistance has been reached
- This 'first barrier' is sensed by an increase in the amount of effort as you move the leg into abduction (Fig. 6.11A)
- Your other (palpating) hand rests passively on the inner thigh, palpating the muscles which are being tested (adductors and medial hamstrings)
- This palpating hand must be in touch with the skin, molded to the contours of the tissues being assessed, but should exert no pressure, and should be completely relaxed
- That palpating hand should also sense the barrier, by virtue of a feeling of increased tension/bind (Fig. 6.11B)
- Normal excursion of the straight leg into abduction is around 45°
- By testing both legs it is possible to evaluate whether the inner thigh muscles are tight and short on both sides, or whether one is and the other is not
- Even if both are tight and short, one may be more restricted than the other. This is the one to treat first using MET
- The point at which the very first sign of bind was noted is the resistance barrier
- Identification and appropriate use of the first sign of resistance (i.e. where bind is first noted) is a fundamental part of the successful use of MET.

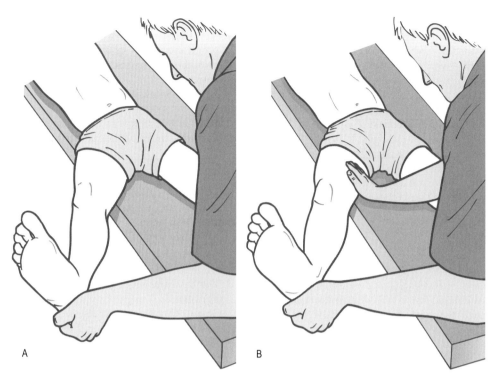

Figure 6.11   (A) Assessment of 'bind'/restriction barrier with the first sign of resistance in the adductors (medial hamstrings) of the right leg. In this example, the practitioner's perception of the transition point, where easy movement alters to demand some degree of effort, is regarded as the barrier. (B) Assessment of 'bind'/restriction barrier with the first sign of resistance in the adductors (medial hamstrings) of the right leg. In this example, the barrier is identified when the palpating hand notes a sense of bind in tissues which were relaxed (at ease) up to that point. (From Chaitow 2001a.)

Treatment of shortness using MET

- The patient is asked to use no more than 20% of available strength to attempt to take the leg gently back towards the table (i.e. to adduct the leg) against firm, unyielding resistance offered by you
- In this example, the patient is trying to take the limb away from the barrier, while you hold the limb firmly (or place yourself between the leg and the table, as in Figure 6.12)
- The patient will be contracting the agonists, the muscles which require release (and which, once released, should allow greater and less restricted abduction)
- The isometric contraction should be introduced slowly, and resisted without any jerking, wobbling, or bouncing
- Maintaining the resistance to the contraction should produce no strain in the therapist
- The contraction should be held for between 7 and 10 s. (This is thought to place 'load' on the Golgi tendon organs, neurologically influencing intrafusal

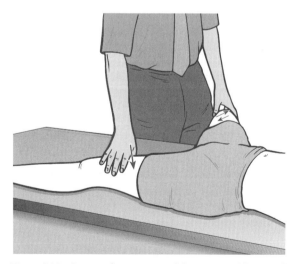

Figure 6.12   Position for treatment of shortness in adductors of the thigh. (From Chaitow 2001a.)

muscle spindle fibers, inhibiting muscle tone and providing the opportunity for the muscle to be taken to a new resting length/resistance barrier without effort; Scariati 1991.)

- An instruction is given to the patient, 'Release your effort, slowly and completely', while the therapist maintains the limb at the same resistance barrier
- The patient is asked to breathe in and out, and to completely relax, and as she exhales, stretch is introduced which takes the tissues to a point just beyond the previous barrier of resistance
- It is useful to have the patient gently assist in taking the (now) relaxed area towards and through the barrier
- The stretch is held for 30 s
- The procedure of contraction, relaxation, followed by patient assisted stretch is repeated (ideally with a rest period between contractions) at least once more.

Reciprocal inhibition (RI)
This example involves abduction of the limb (i.e. shortened adductors), against resistance.

- The barrier, first sense of restriction/bind, is evaluated as the limb is abducted, at which point the limb is returned a fraction towards a mid-range position (by a few degrees only)
- From this position, the patient is asked to attempt to abduct the leg, using no more than 20% of strength, taking it towards the restriction barrier, while the therapist resists this effort
- After 7 s, following the end of the contraction, the patient is asked to 'release and relax', followed by inhalation and exhalation and further relaxation, at which time the limb is guided through the new barrier, with the patient's assistance.
- This stretch is held for at least 30 s.

MET: some common errors and contraindications

Greenman (1996) summarizes several of the important elements of MET as follows.
There is a patient-active muscle contraction:

- from a controlled position
- in a specific direction
- met by therapist-applied distinct counterforce
- involving a controlled intensity of contraction.

Patient errors during MET usage
Commonly based on inadequate instruction from the therapist.

1 Contraction is too strong (*remedy*: give specific guidelines, e.g. 'use only 20% of strength', or whatever is more appropriate)

2 Contraction is in the wrong direction (*remedy*: give simple but accurate instructions)
3 Contraction is not sustained for long enough (*remedy*: instruct the patient to hold the contraction until told to ease off, and give an idea ahead of time as to how long this will be)
4 The patient does not relax completely after the contraction (*remedy*: have them release and relax, and then inhale and exhale once or twice, with the suggestion 'now relax completely').

Therapist errors in application of MET
1 Inaccurate control of position of joint or muscle in relation to the resistance barrier (*remedy*: have a clear image of what is required and apply it)
2 Inadequate counterforce to the contraction (*remedy*: meet and match the force)
3 Counterforce is applied in an inappropriate direction (*remedy*: ensure precise direction needed for best results)
4 Moving to a new position too hastily after the contraction (take your time to have the patient relax completely before moving to a new position)
5 Inadequate patient instruction is given (*remedy*: get the instructions right so that the patient can cooperate)
6 The therapist fails to maintain the stretch position for a period of time that allows soft tissues to begin to lengthen (ideally 30 s, but certainly not just a few seconds).

Contraindications and side-effects of MET

- If pathology is suspected, no MET should be used until an accurate diagnosis has been established
- Pathology (osteoporosis, arthritis, etc.) does not rule out the use of MET, but its presence needs to be established so that dosage of application can be modified accordingly (amount of effort used, number of repetitions, stretching introduced or not, etc.)
- There are no other contraindications except for the injunction to cause no pain.

Pulsed MET

There is another MET variation, which is powerful and useful: pulsed MET (Ruddy 1962). This simple method has been found to be very useful since it effectively accomplishes a number of changes at the same time, involving the local nerve supply, improved circulation and oxygenation of tissues, reduction of contraction, etc.

This method depends for its effectiveness on the 'pulsed' efforts of the person producing them being very light indeed, with no 'wobble' or 'bounce', just the barest activation of the muscles involved.

An example of self-applied pulsed MET:

- Sit at a table, rest your elbows on it, and tilt your head forwards as far as it will go comfortably and rest your hands against your forehead
- Use a pulsing rhythm of pressure of your head pushing against your *firm* hand contact, involving about 2 pulsations per second (against your hands) for 10 s
- After 20 pulsations, re-test the range of forward bending of your neck. It should go much further, more easily than before
- This method will have relaxed the muscles of the region, especially those involved in flexion, and will have produced 20 small reciprocal inhibition 'messages' to the muscles on the back of your neck which were preventing easy flexion
- Pulsed MET may be used for restricted muscles or joints in any part of the body
- The simple rule is to have the patient engage the restriction barrier, while you provide a point of resistance (with your hands) as the patient pulses towards the barrier rhythmically
- No pain should be felt
- After 20 contractions in 10 s, the barrier should have retreated and the process can be repeated from the new barrier
- The pulsing method should always be against a fixed resistance, just as in other MET methods.

MET methods for key muscles that have been identified as short are given in Chapter 7.

POSITIONAL RELEASE TECHNIQUE (PRT)

PRT is itself made up of a number of quite different methods, but the one that is probably most suitable for use in a massage therapy context is called strain/counterstrain (SCS). In order to understand this method, a brief explanation is needed (Chaitow 2003b, D'Ambrogio & Roth 1997, Deig 2001). Jones (1981) described the evolution of strain/counterstrain as depending upon identification of 'tender' points found in the soft tissues associated with joints that have been stretched, strained or traumatized.

- These tender points are usually located in soft tissues shortened at the time of the strain or trauma (i.e. in the antagonists to those that were stretched during the process of injury)
- For example, in spinal problems following on from a forward-bending strain, in which back pain is complained of, the appropriate 'tender' point

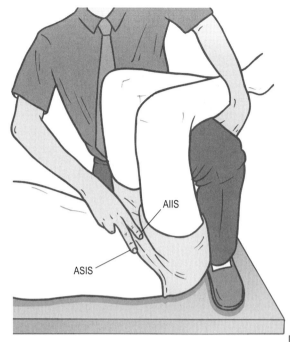

Figure 6.13   Position of ease for flexion strain of T9 to lower lumbar regions involves flexion, side-bending and rotation until ease is achieved in monitored tender point on the lower abdominal wall or the ASIS area.

will be found on the anterior surface of the body (Fig. 6.13)

- The same process of tender point development in shortened structures takes place in response to chronic adaptation
- Tender points are exquisitely sensitive on palpation but usually painless otherwise
- Once identified, such points are used as monitors (explained below) as the area, or the whole body, is repositioned ('fine tuned') until the palpated pain disappears or reduces substantially
- Tissue tension almost always eases at the same time as the easing of pain in the palpated point, making it possible to palpate the person, or part, into an ease position
- If the 'position of ease' is held for some 90 s, there is often a resolution of the dysfunction which resulted from the trauma.

Positional release exercise

- Using one of the skin assessment methods discussed earlier in this chapter, or NMT, or whatever palpation method you are used to using, palpate the musculotendinous tissues that are antagonists to those that were being stretched during a joint or

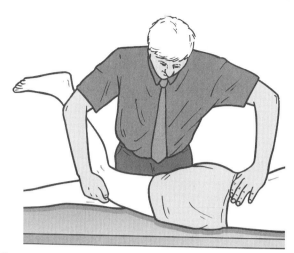

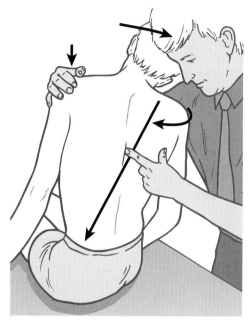

Figure 6.14 Position of ease for a tender point associated with an extension strain of the lumbar strain involves use of the legs of the prone patient as means of achieving extension and fine-tuning.

spinal trauma or strain, or which are chronically shortened as part of a longstanding problem

- The area being assessed should be one that is not being complained of as being painful
- Any localized, unusually tender area in such tissue can be used as a 'tender point'
- You should apply sufficient pressure to that point to cause mild discomfort and then slowly position the joint or area in such a way as to remove the tenderness from the point (Figs 6.14, 6.15)
- Creating 'ease' in the tissues housing the point usually involves producing some degree of increased slack in the palpated tissues
- Hold this position for 90 s and then slowly return to a neutral position and re-palpate
- The tenderness should have reduced or vanished, and functionality should be improved.

Main features of PRT

- All movements should be passive (therapist controls the movement, patient does nothing), and movements are painless, slow and deliberate
- Existing pain reduces, and no additional or new pain is created
- Movement is *away* from restriction barriers
- Muscle origins and insertions are brought together, rather than being stretched
- Movement is away from any direction, or position, that causes pain or discomfort
- Tissues being palpated relax
- Painful tissues being palpated (possibly a trigger point) reduce in pain

Figure 6.15 Treatment of thoracic region dysfunction (in this example 'tissue tension' to the right of the 6th thoracic vertebrae). One hand monitors tissue status as the patient is asked to 'sit straight' and to then slightly extend the spine. The operator then introduces compression from the right shoulder towards the left hip which automatically produces sidebending and rotation to the right. If ease is noted in the palpated tissues, the position is held for 30–90 seconds.

- It is often the case that the position of ease is a replica of a position of strain that started whatever problem the patient now has.

Guidelines for PRT use

1 For treatment of tender points on the anterior surface of the body, flexion, sidebending and rotation should be *towards* the palpated point, followed by fine-tuning to reduce sensitivity by at least 70%

2 For treatment of tender points on the posterior surface of the body, extension, sidebending and rotation should be *away* from the palpated point, followed by fine tuning to reduce sensitivity by 70%

3 The closer the tender point is to the midline, the less sidebending and rotation should be required, and the further from the midline, the more sidebending and rotation should be required, in order to effect ease and comfort in the tender point (without any additional pain or discomfort being produced anywhere else)

4   The direction towards which sidebending is introduced when trying to find a position of ease often needs to be away from the side of the palpated pain point, especially in relation to tender points found on the posterior aspect of the body.

The SCS process described step-by-step

- To use the strain/counterstrain (SCS) approach a painful point is located
- This can be a 'tender' point, or an actual trigger point
- Sufficient pressure is applied to the point to cause some pain
- If it is a trigger point ensure that just enough pressure is being applied to cause the referred symptoms
- The patient is told to give the pain being felt a value of '10'

Note: This is not a situation in which the patient is asked to ascribe a pain level out of 10, instead it is one in which the question asked is 'Does the pressure hurt?'

If the answer is 'Yes', then the patient is told: 'Give the level of pain you are now feeling a value of 10, and as I move the area around and ask for feedback, give me the new pain level – whatever it is'.

- It is important to ask the patient to avoid comments such as 'The pain is increasing' or 'It's getting less', or any other verbal comment, other than *a number out of 10*. This helps to avoid undue delay in the process
- In this example, we can imagine that the tender, or trigger, point is in the gluteus medius (Fig. 6.16)
- The patient would be prone, and the therapist would be applying sufficient pressure to the point

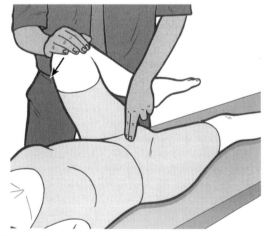

Figure 6.16   Treatment of pubococcygeus dysfunction.

in the gluteus medius to register pain which he/she would be told has a value of '10'
- The supported leg on the side of pain would be moved in one direction (say extension at the hip) as the patient is asked to give a value out of 10 for the pain
- If the pain reduces, another direction might be introduced (say adduction) – and the question is repeated
- If the pain increases, a different movement direction would be chosen
- By gradually working through all the movement possibilities, in various directions, and possibly adding compression and distraction, a position would be found where pain drops by at least 70% (i.e. the score reaches '3', or less)
- Once this 'position of ease' has been found, after all the careful slow-motion fine-tuning, it is maintained for not less than 90 s – and sometimes more – after which a slow return is made to the starting position
- Range of motion, and degree of previous pain should have changed for the better.

In different tissues, the possible directions of movement might include flexion, extension, rotation one way or the other, side flexion one way or the other, translation (shunting, or evaluating joint-play) as well as compression or distraction – to find the position of maximum ease.

What happens when tissues are at ease?
What happens when tissues are at ease (whether 90 s or much longer)?

1   Pain receptors (nociceptors) reduce in sensitivity, something that is of importance where pain is a feature, whether this involves trigger points or not (Bailey & Dick 1992, Van Buskirk 1990)
2   In the comfort/ease position there is a marked improvement in blood flow and oxygenation through the tissues
3   Facilitated areas (spinal or trigger points) will be less active, less sensitized, calmer and less painful.

Positional release is used as part of the integrated neuromuscular inhibition (INIT) sequence described below, for trigger point deactivation.

INTEGRATED NEUROMUSCULAR INHIBITION (FOR TRIGGER POINT DEACTIVATION)

An integrated treatment sequence has been developed for the deactivation of myofascial trigger points. The method is as follows:

1   The trigger point is identified by palpation.

2   Ischemic compression is applied in either a sustained or intermittent manner.

3   When referred or local pain starts to reduce in intensity, the compression treatment stops.

4   The patient should be told, e.g.:

'I am going to press that same point again, and I want you to give the pain that you feel a 'value' of 10. I will then gently reposition the area and you will feel differences in the levels of pain. In some positions the pain may increase, in others it will decrease. When I ask you for feedback as to what's happening to the pain, please give me a number out of 10. If the pain has increased it may go up – to say 11 or 12. Just give me the number you are feeling. We are aiming to find a position in which the pain drops to 3 or less, and the more accurately you give me the 'pain score' the faster I will be able to fine-tune the process, so that we can get to the 'comfort position'.

5   Using these methods (as described in the section above, on Positional Release Technique) the tissues housing the trigger point are then carefully placed in a position of ease.

6   This ease position is held for approximately 20–30 s, to allow neurological resetting, reduction in pain receptor activity, and enhanced local circulation/oxygenation.

7   An isometric contraction is then focused into the musculature around the trigger point to create post isometric relaxation (PIR), as discussed in the MET section earlier in this chapter.

8   The way this is done varies with the particular part of the body being treated. Sometimes all that is necessary is to say to the patient, 'Tighten the muscles around the place where my thumb is pressing'.

9   At other times, if the patient is being supported in a position of ease, it may be helpful to say something like: 'I am going to let go of your leg (or neck, or arm, or whatever else you are supporting) and I want you to hold the position on your own for a few seconds'. In one way or another you need to induce a contraction of the muscle tissues surrounding the trigger point, so that they can be more easily stretched afterwards.

10   After the contraction (5–7 s, with the patient using only a small amount of effort), the soft tissues housing the trigger point are stretched locally (Fig. 6.17A,B).

11   The local stretch is important because it is often the case in a large muscle that stretching the whole muscle will effectively lengthen it, but the tight bundle where the trigger point is situated will be relatively un-stretched, like a knot in a piece of elastic which remains knotted even though the elastic is held at stretch.

12   After holding the local stretch for approximately 30 s, the entire muscle should then be contracted and stretched – again holding that stretch for at least 30 s.

13   The patient should assist in stretching movements (whenever possible) by activating the antagonists and so facilitating the stretch.

14   A towel that has been wrung out in warm/hot water placed over the treated tissues for 5 min helps to ease the soreness that may follow this treatment.

15   Within 24 h, the trigger should have reduced in activity considerably, or no longer be active.

16   Re-testing immediately after the INIT sequence may not offer evidence of this, as tissues will be tender.

SPRAY-AND-STRETCH METHODS

An effective method for deactivation of trigger points, and also for easing pain and releasing chronic muscle spasm, is use of spray-and-stretch methods (Mennell 1975).

- A container of vapocoolant spray with a calibrated nozzle that delivers a fine jet stream, or a source of ice, is needed
- The jet stream should have sufficient force to carry in the air for at least 3 ft. A mist-like spray is less desirable (Fig. 6.18A,B)
- Ice can consist of a cylinder of ice formed by freezing water in a paper cup and then peeling this off the ice. A wooden handle will have been frozen into the ice to allow for its ease of application, as it is rolled from the trigger towards the referred area in a series of sweeps
- A piece of ice may also be used, directly against the skin, for the same purpose, although this tends to be messy as the ice melts
- Whichever method is chosen, the patient should be comfortably supported to promote muscular relaxation
- If a spray is used, the container is held about 2 ft away, in such a manner that the jet stream meets the body surface at an acute angle or at a tangent, not perpendicularly. This lessens the shock of the impact
- The stream/ice massage is applied in one direction, not back and forth
- Each sweep is started at the trigger point and is moved slowly and evenly outward over the reference

Figure 6.17 (A) 'S' bend pressure applied to tense or fibrotic musculature. (B) The lower trapezius fibers are treated in the same way.

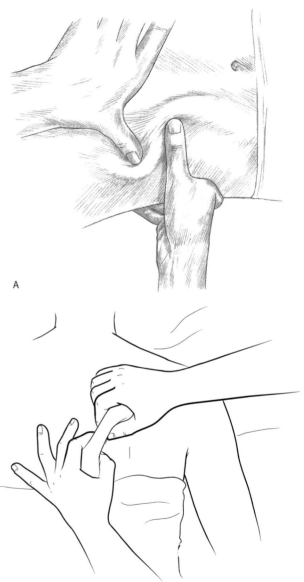

A

B

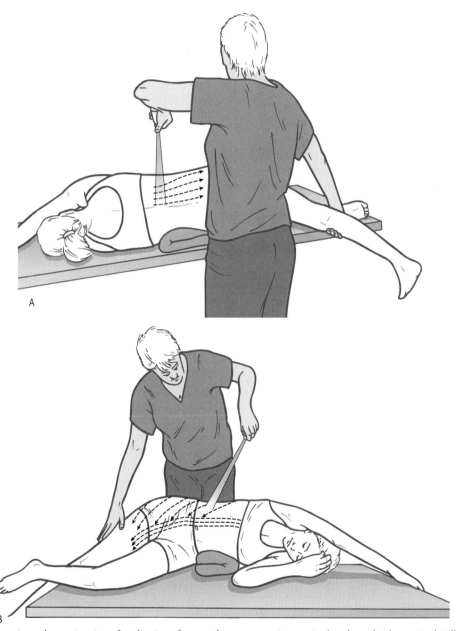

Figure 6.18 Anterior and posterior view of application of vapocoolant spray to trigger point (quadratus lumborum in this illustration). Muscles housing trigger points are placed at stretch while a coolant spray is utilized to chill the point and the area between it and the target reference area.

zone. The direction of chilling should be in line with the muscle fibers towards their insertion
- The optimum speed of movement of the sweep/roll over the skin seems to be about 4 in (10 cm) per s
- Each sweep is started slightly proximal to the trigger point and is moved slowly and evenly through the reference zone to cover it and extend slightly beyond it
- These sweeps are repeated in a rhythm of a few seconds on and a few seconds off, until all the skin over trigger and reference areas has been covered once or twice
- If aching or 'cold pain' develops, or if the application of the spray/ice sets off a reference of pain, the interval between applications is lengthened
- Care must be taken not to frost or blanch the skin
- During the application of cold or directly after it, the taut fibers should be stretched passively
- The fibers should not be stretched in advance of the cold
- Steady, gentle stretching is usually essential if a satisfactory result is to be achieved
- As relaxation of the muscle occurs, continued stretch should be maintained for 20–30 s, and after each series of cold applications active motion is tested
- An attempt should be made to restore the full range of motion, but always within the limits of pain, as sudden overstretching can increase existing muscle spasm
- The entire procedure may occupy 15–20 min and should not be rushed. The importance of re-establishing normal motion in conjunction with the use of the chilling is well founded.

REHABILITATION EXERCISE METHODS

Norris (1999) advises the following guidelines for re-establishing back stability, using stabilization exercises for the different triage groups:

- *Simple backache*: Begin stability exercises and continue until fully functional
- *Nerve root compression*: Begin exercise as pain allows, but refer to specialist if there has been no improvement within 4 weeks
- *Serious pathology*: Use back stabilization exercises only after surgical or medical intervention.

There are many interlocking rehabilitation features (Liebenson 1996) that may be involved in any particular case:

- normalization of soft tissue dysfunction
- deactivation of myofascial trigger points

- strengthening weakened structures
- proprioceptive reeducation using physical therapy methods
- postural and breathing reeducation
- ergonomic, nutritional and stress management strategies
- psychotherapy, counseling or pain management techniques
- occupational therapy which specializes in activating healthy coping mechanisms
- appropriate exercise strategies to overcome deconditioning.

A team approach to rehabilitation is called for where referral and cooperation between healthcare professionals allow the best outcome to be achieved. You are encouraged to develop an understanding of the multiple disciplines with which you can interface so that the best outcome for the patient can be achieved.

Core stability and breathing rehabilitation exercises are described in Chapter 8.

MASSAGE

A variety of massage applications can be employed to accompany the methods outlined in this chapter. The primary massage techniques include:

- Effluerage
- Petrissage
- Kneading
- Inhibition pressure
- Vibration and friction
- Transverse friction.

Massage effects explained

A combination of physical effects occur, apart from the undoubted anxiety-reducing (Sandler 1983) influences that involve biochemical changes. Among the many effects of massage techniques are the following examples:

- Plasma cortisol and catecholamine concentrations alter markedly as anxiety levels drop and depression is also reduced (Field 1992)
- Serotonin levels rise as sleep is enhanced, even in severely ill patients – preterm infants, cancer patients and people with irritable bowel problems as well as HIV-positive individuals (Acolet 1993, Ferel-Torey 1993, Xujian 1990)
- Pressure strokes tend to displace fluid content, encouraging venous, lymphatic and tissue drainage

- Increase of blood flow results in fresh oxygenated blood which aids in normalization via increased capillary filtration and venous capillary pressure
- Edema is reduced and so are the effects of pain-inducing substances which may be present
- Decreases occur in the sensitivity of the gamma efferent control of the muscle spindles thereby reducing any shortening tendency of the muscles (Puustjarvi 1990)

- A transition occurs in the ground substance of fascia (the colloidal matrix) from gel to sol which increases internal hydration and assists in the removal of toxins from the tissue (Oschman 1997)
- Pressure techniques can have a direct effect on the Golgi tendon organs, which detect the load applied to the tendon or muscle.

KEY POINTS

- Good palpation skills allow a therapist to rapidly and accurately localize and identify dysfunctional tissues
- Neuromuscular technique (NMT) offers a unique way of searching tissues for local changes (such as trigger points) in a sequential way, and then treating whatever is located
- Muscle energy techniques (MET) offer useful ways of encouraging length into previously tight, short, soft tissues
- Positional release technique (PRT) offers painless ways for encouraging release of hypertonicity and spasm

- Sprain-and-stretch chilling methods are of proven value in trigger point deactivation and easing spasm
- Integrated neuromuscular inhibition (INIT) is a sequence involving pressure methods, together with MET and PRT for trigger point deactivation
- Rehabilitation exercise methods are vital for ultimate recovery and prevention
- Massage combines with any of these approaches and has unique attributes of its own in back pain care.

References

Acolet D 1993 Changes in plasma cortisol and catecholamine concentrations on response to massage in preterm infants. Archives of Diseases in Childhood 68:29–31

Adams T, Steinmetz M, Heisey S et al 1982 Physiologic basis for skin properties in palpatory physical diagnosis. Journal of the American Osteopathic Association 81(6):366–377

Bailey M, Dick L 1992 Nociceptive considerations in treating with counterstrain. Journal of the American Osteopathic Association 92:334–341

Ballantyne F, Fryer G, McLaughlin P 2003 The effect of muscle energy technique on hamstring extensibility: the mechanism of altered flexibility. Journal of Osteopathic Medicine 6(2):59–63

Bischof I, Elmiger G. 1960 Connective tissue massage. In: Licht S (ed.) Massage, manipulation and traction. Licht, New Haven

Chaitow L 2001a Muscle energy techniques, 2nd edn. Churchill Livingstone, Edinburgh

Chaitow L 2001b Positional release techniques, 2nd edn. Churchill Livingstone, Edinburgh

Chaitow L 2003a Modern neuromuscular techniques, 2nd edn. Churchill Livingstone, Edinburgh, p 120–131

Chaitow L 2003b Positional release techniques, 2nd edn. Churchill Livingstone, Edinburgh

Chaitow L, DeLany J 2000 Clinical applications of neuromuscular technique, Volume 1. Churchill Livingstone, Edinburgh

Cohen J, Gibbons R 1998 Raymond Nimmo and the evolution of trigger point therapy. Journal of Manipulation and Physiological Therapeutics 21(3):167–172

D'Ambrogio K, Roth G 1997 Positional release therapy. Mosby, St Louis

Deig D 2001 Positional release technique. Butterworth-Heinemann, Boston

Ferel-Torey A 1993 Use of therapeutic massage as a nursing intervention to modify anxiety and perceptions of cancer pain. Cancer Nursing 16(2):93–101

Field T 1992 Massage reduces depression and anxiety in child and adolescent psychiatry patients. Journal of the American Academy of Adolescent Psychiatry 31:125–131

Gibbons P, Tehan P 2001 Spinal manipulation: indications, risks and benefits. Churchill Livingstone, Edinburgh

Goodridge J, Kuchera W 1997 Muscle energy treatment techniques. In: Ward R (ed.) Foundations of osteopathic medicine. Williams and Wilkins, Baltimore

Greenman P 1996 Principles of manual medicine, 2nd edn. Williams and Wilkins, Baltimore

Janda V 1978 Muscles, central nervous motor regulation, and back problems. In: Korr IM (ed.) Neurobiologic mechanisms in manipulative therapy. Plenum, New York

Jones L 1981 Strain and counterstrain. Academy of Applied Osteopathy, Colorado Springs

Kappler R 1997 Palpatory skills. In: Ward R (ed.) Foundations for osteopathic medicine. Williams &Wilkins, Baltimore

Lewit K 1996 Role of manipulation in spinal rehabilitation. In: Liebenson C (ed.) Rehabilitation of the spine. Williams and Wilkins, Baltimore

Lewit K 1999 Manipulative therapy in rehabilitation of the locomotor system, 3rd edn. Butterworths, London

Liebenson C (ed.) 1996 Rehabilitation of the spine. Williams and Wilkins, Baltimore

Maitland G 2001 Maitland's vertebral manipulation, 6th edn. Butterworth Heinemann, Oxford

Mennell J 1975 Therapeutic use of cold. Journal of the American Osteopathic Association 74(12):1146–1158

Norris C M 1999 Functional load abdominal training. Journal of Bodywork and Movement Therapies 3(3):150–158

Oschman J L 1997 What is healing energy? Part 5: Gravity, structure, and emotions. Journal of Bodywork and Movement Therapies 1(5):307–308

Petty N, Moore A 1998 Neuromusculoskeletal examination and assessment. Churchill Livingstone, Edinburgh

Puustjarvi K 1990 Effects of massage in patients with chronic tension headaches. Acupuncture and Electrotherapeutics Research 15:159–162

Reed B, Held J 1988 Effects of sequential connective tissue massage on autonomic nervous system of middle-aged and elderly adults. Physical Therapy 68(8):1231–1234

Rowlands A V, Marginson V F, Lee J 2003 Chronic flexibility gains: effect of isometric contraction duration during proprioceptive neuromuscular facilitation stretching techniques. Research Quarterly Exercise & Sport 74(1):47–51

Ruddy T J 1962 Osteopathic rapid rhythmic resistive technic. Academy of Applied Osteopathy Yearbook, Carmel, p 23–31

Sandler S 1983 The physiology of soft tissue massage. British Osteopathic Journal 15:1–6

Scariati P 1991 Myofascial release concepts. In: DiGiovanna E (ed.) An osteopathic approach to diagnosis and treatment. Lippincott, London

Stone C 1999 Science in the art of osteopathy. Stanley Thornes, Cheltenham UK

Van Buskirk R 1990 Nociceptive reflexes and the somatic dysfunction. Journal of the American Osteopathic Association 90:792–809

Ward R 1997 Foundations of osteopathic medicine. Williams and Wilkins, Baltimore

Xujian S 1990 Effects of massage and temperature on permeability of initial lymphatics. Lymphology 23:48–50

Youngs B 1962 Physiological basis of neuro-muscular technique. British Naturopathic Journal 5(6):176–190

Chapter 7

Outcome based massage

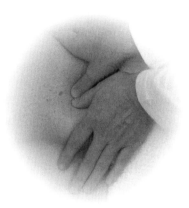

INTRODUCTION

The information up to this point has involved both theory and methodology specifically focused to understanding, assessing, determining appropriateness of treatment and finally developing massage treatment approaches for low back pain.

This chapter specifically concerns the integration of theory, assessment and treatment of low back pain into general massage application and will not repeat assessment and treatment recommendations.

The focus of this chapter is to describe ways of incorporating the information and skills outlined in previous chapters into a massage session, so that the essence of the full body massage experience remains and is enhanced by the ability to specifically address low back dysfunction in the context of massage. Massage can provide an integrated approach for treatment of low back pain addressing many of the major factors already discussed.

When massage is used to address a specific problem or set of symptoms it is considered outcome based massage. *Outcome based massage* relies on results instead of methods and modalities. Various massage methods can be combined to achieve outcomes. For example, if a massage therapist is working with a multidisciplinary healthcare team to treat low back problems, outcome based instructions to the massage therapist might include suggestions such as:

- increase lumbo-dorsal fascia pliability
- lengthen shortened hamstrings
- address trigger point referred pain from the psoas muscle
- reduce sympathetic arousal.

The instructions are unlikely to be: 'apply Swedish massage with reflexology and energy based modalities'.

While the difference between massage modalities and massage based on outcome goals may seem simple, this is actually a major paradigm shift that the massage community continues to grapple with. Approaching therapeutic massage to address low back pain needs to be outcome based, since different massage modalities can be used alone, or in combination, and with other methods to achieve a positive change for those experiencing back pain and stiffness.

To be proficient in outcome based massage it is necessary to be skilled in evaluation and clinical reasoning in order to develop appropriate treatment plans. The information in previous chapters provides the foundation upon which the massage therapist can make appropriate treatment plan decisions in the context of treating back pain problems.

It is possible to include much of the assessment process into a general full body massage session. In fact it is desirable to consider the first few massage sessions as assessment. Then, based on assessment information gathered during massage sessions, coupled with other information from a comprehensive history, tests performed outside the context of massage, together with information from other professionals involved with the patient, a specific treatment plan can be developed to achieve the outcome goals.

Because most people have preconceived ideas about what a massage should be (relaxing, passive, general) it becomes important to incorporate both assessment and treatment into the massage in such a way that the generalized full body experience of the massage is not compromised. People enjoy massage because it feels good, and is a nurturing integrated experience. This major strength of massage needs to be preserved, not replaced. General non-specific full body massage, based on the outcomes of decreased sympathetic arousal and maladaptive stress response, tactile pleasure sensation and nurturing, is effective in the treatment of low back symptoms even if nothing else is done (Yates 2004). It is prudent to preserve these qualities and benefits of massage when addressing specific conditions such as low back dysfunction.

The massage therapist can increase the effectiveness of massage treatment by becoming more skilled in how to target a specific outcome, such as reducing pain and stiffness in the low back. This is accomplished by incorporating assessment skills and targeted treatment methods based on that assessment information into the full body massage session. Targeted treatment such as for deactivation of trigger points can feel intense and/or uncomfortable. These methods are often better accepted and integrated by the patient when 'wrapped' in the pleasure and nurturing experience of a general massage session. Since low back problems are so common and massage has been shown to be beneficial (see Ch. 1), the massage therapist needs to be skilled in this area.

The low back pain and dysfunction targeted in this text is non-specific, mechanical. It is typically a cumulative response to many different factors such as: postural distortion, a combination of short soft tissue and long weak muscles or lax ligaments, various types of joint dysfunction especially instability, generalized stress and breathing dysfunction, repetitive strain, lack of movement, and so on.

Based on many years of professional experience, client populations that typically seek massage are often prone to back ache. These populations include athletes, and anyone who works in the sport massage area needs to understand the predisposing factors, assessment and treatment of low back pain. Those involved with rehabilitation exercise for cardiovascular conditions or weight management, or in physical therapy receiving care for a variety of physical injuries can develop secondary muscular back pain from the stress and altered movement of the exercises (Wieting et al 2005).

It is logical that individuals undergoing medical procedures such as surgery may develop back pain secondary to the positioning required to perform the procedure, extended bed rest, reduced physical activity, anxiety and other predisposing factors (see Ch. 1 for more on these issues). Back pain is a major treatment concern in healthcare in many populations and includes 'growing pains' in children and adolescents, postural distortion during pregnancy, postural strain from obesity, and muscle pain as part of osteoporosis and other conditions related to aging (Yates 2004).

Management of low back pain and improvement in function requires life-style changes on the part of the client/patient and compliance with various treatment protocols. Unfortunately, many people are not diligent when it comes to implementing these changes. For these individuals low back pain can frequently be symptomatically managed with massage. This means that the massage outcome goal is pain management, more so than targeting a change in the factors causing the condition. And just as pain medication will wear off, so will the effects of massage, so it may need to be more frequent in order to maintain symptom management.

Massage may actually be the treatment of choice for those people who will not be compliant with a multi-disciplinary care plan for low back dysfunction. Based on the assumption that they are not going to make behavioral changes, or do the necessary exercises, massage can replace – to some extent – the activities necessary to maintain pliability and flexibility in shortened soft tissue structures as well as reducing generalized stress. People can become discouraged, which increases the tendency to be non-compliant with self-treatment protocols. A massage twice a week can often manage the pain and dysfunction in these people by moving fluids, lengthening short structures, stimulating internal pain modulating mechanisms, and by reducing generalized motor tone by decreasing sympathetic autonomic nervous system activity, as well as by providing pleasurable relaxation experiences.

The goal is not to 'fix' the back pain but to both mask it and superimpose short-term beneficial changes in the tissue. If these patients were treated with medication they would take muscle relaxants, some sort of analgesic and anti-inflammatory, and possibly mood modulating drugs. All of these medications have potentially serious side-effects with long-term use, making them undesirable in the management of chronic back pain. Massage may accomplish similar results to those achieved by medication, if applied frequently and consistently, and without the side-effect problem. Massage can replace or help reduce the dose of various medications, and it can be used indefinitely to treat the symptoms of chronic back dysfunction. Massage has few if any side-effects, is cost effective, produces at least short-term benefits and since people typically enjoy massage they tend to be compliant about attending sessions (Fritz 2004). This situation is not ideal but it is not the worst-case situation either, and it is possible that eventually the patient/client will reach a point in their life when they are able and willing to be more responsible for the life-style and attitude changes necessary to manage chronic back pain and dysfunction.

DESCRIBING MASSAGE

There is an evolution taking place in massage. The shift from a modality focus (examples: Swedish massage, reflexology, deep tissue massage, Amma, Lomi Lomi), to an outcome focus requires a change in terminology and how massage application is described. One definition of massage is that it represents the manual manipulation of the soft tissues. Soft tissue manipulations create various mechanical forces which cause shifts in the form and function of the body. The physiological responses of the body to massage are not specific to the modality used, but to what is described as qualities of touch.

Qualities of touch

Massage application involves touching the body to manipulate the soft tissue, influence body fluid movement and stimulate neuroendocrine responses. How the physical contact is applied is considered by the qualities of touch. Based on information from massage pioneer Gertrude Beard and current trends in therapeutic massage, the massage application can be described as follows (De Domenico & Wood 1997).

Depth of pressure

- Depth of pressure (Fig. 7.1) (compressive force) which is extremely important can be light, moderate, deep, or variable
- Most soft tissue areas of the body consist of three to five layers of tissue, including: the skin; the superficial fascia; the superficial, middle, and deep layers of muscle; and the various fascial sheaths and connective tissue structures
- Pressure should be delivered through each successive layer to reach the deeper layers without damage and discomfort to the more superficial tissues
- The deeper the pressure, the broader the base of contact required on the surface of the body
- It takes more pressure to address thick, dense tissue than delicate, thin tissue
- Depth of pressure is important for both assessment and treatment of soft tissue dysfunctions
- Soft tissue dysfunction can form in all layers of tissue

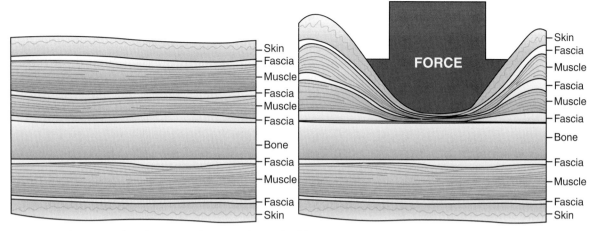

Figure 7.1 Compressive force. (From Fritz S 2004 Fundamentals of therapeutic massage, 3rd edn. Mosby, St Louis.)

- In order to treat various changes in soft tissue (such as a trigger point), it is necessary to be able to apply the correct level of pressure to both reach the location of the point and compress the tissue to alter flow of circulation
- Soft tissue dysfunctions located in surface tissue require less depth of pressure than those located in deeper muscle layers.

Drag

- Drag (Fig. 7.2) describes the amount of pull (stretch) on the tissue (tensile force)
- Drag is applicable for various types of palpation assessment for soft tissue dysfunctions, including skin drag assessment and functional technique used to identify areas of ease and bind
- *Ease* is identified when tissue moves freely and easily while *bind* is where tissue palpates as stuck, leathery or thick
- Drag is also a component of connective tissue methods used to treat soft tissue dysfunctions and lymphatic drainage methods.

Direction

- Direction can move from the center of the body out (centrifugal) or in from the extremities towards the center of the body (centripetal)
- Direction can proceed from proximal to distal (or vice versa) of the muscle, following the muscle fibers, transverse to the tissue fibers, or in circular motions
- Direction is a factor in stretching tissues containing soft tissue dysfunctions or in the methods that influence blood and lymphatic fluid movement.

Speed

- Speed is the rate at which massage methods are applied
- The speed can be fast, slow, or variable depending on the demands of the tissues being addressed and the state of the client/patient (faster more energizing in situations where stimulation is called for, slower and more rhythmic where calming influences are needed).

Rhythm

- Rhythm refers to the regularity of application of the technique
- If the method is applied at regular intervals, it is considered even, or rhythmic
- If the method is disjointed or irregular, it is considered uneven, or arrhythmic
- The on/off aspect of compression applied to a trigger point to encourage circulation to the area should be rhythmic, as should lymphatic drainage application
- Jostling and shaking can be rhythmic or arrhythmic.

Frequency

- Frequency is the rate at which the method is repeated in a given time-frame
- This aspect of massage relates to how often the treatment, such as ischemic compression or gliding, is performed
- In general, the massage practitioner repeats each method about three times before moving or switching to a different approach

Figure 7.2   Drag. (From Fritz S 2004 Fundamentals of therapeutic massage, 3rd edn. Mosby, St Louis.)

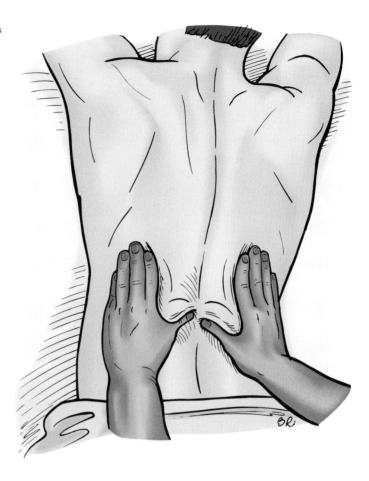

- The first application can be considered as assessment, the second as treatment, and the third as post assessment
- If the post assessment indicates remaining dysfunction, then the frequency is increased to repeat the treatment/post assessment application.

Duration

- Duration is the length of time that the method lasts, or that the manipulation stays focused on the same location
- Typically, duration of a specific method is approximately 60 s, although functional methods that position the tissue or joint in the ease (the way it wants to move) or bind (the way it does not want to move) can be an exception and may need to be applied for longer periods
- Duration relates to how long compression is applied to soft tissue areas of dysfunction, or how long a stretch is held.

The following example demonstrates how some of these qualities can be used to describe a massage modality. Myofascial/connective tissue methods (Fig. 7.3) may be indicated in the management and treatment of low back pain.

Massage used to influence superficial fascia can be explained as follows: light pressure, with sustained drag, to create tension forces, stretching the tissues just past their end of range barriers (bind) in multiple directions, for a duration of 60 s and repeated three times.

DELIVERY OF MASSAGE

- Through these varied qualities of touch, delivery of massage methods can be adapted to achieve the outcomes best suited to meet the needs of the client
- The mode of application (e.g. gliding/effleurage, kneading/pétrissage, compression) provides the most efficient way to apply the methods
- Each method can be varied, depending on the desired outcome, by adjusting depth, drag, direction, speed, rhythm, frequency and duration

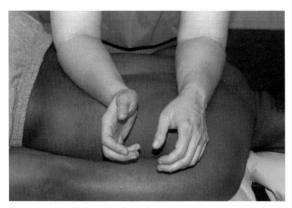

Figure 7.3 Application of myofascial/connective tissue methods demonstrating drag and tension force. (Reproduced with kind permission from Mosby's Massage Career Development Series 2006.)

- In perfecting massage application, the quality of touch is as important as the method
- Quality of touch is altered when there is a contraindication or caution for massage
- For example, when a person is fatigued, the duration of the application should be reduced; if a client has a fragile bone structure, the depth of pressure should be altered.

Components of massage methods

- All massage methods introduce forces into the soft tissues
- These forces stimulate various physiologic responses
- Some massage applications are more mechanical than others
- Connective tissue and fluid dynamics are most affected by mechanical force.

Connective tissue is influenced by mechanical forces by changing its pliability, orientation and length (Yahia et al 1993).

- The movement of fluids in the body is a mechanical process, for example the mechanical pumping of the heart
- Forces applied to the body mimic various pumping mechanisms of the heart, arteries, veins, lymphatics, muscles, respiratory system and digestive tract (Lederman 1997)
- Neuroendocrine stimulation occurs when forces are applied during massage that generate various shifts in physiology (NCCAM 2004)
- Massage causes the release of vasodilators, substances that then increase circulation in an area

- Massage stimulates the relaxation response reducing sympathetic autonomic nervous system dominance (Freeman & Lawlis 2001)
- Forces applied during massage stimulate proprioceptors which alter motor tone in muscles (Lederman 1997)
- Typically these two responses to massage (fluid dynamics and neuroendocrine) occur together, although the intent of the massage application can target one response more than the other.

Different forces

It is helpful to identify the different types of mechanical forces and to understand the ways in which mechanical forces applied during massage act therapeutically on the body. The forces created by massage are tension loading, compression loading, bending loading, shear loading, rotation or torsion loading and combined loading. How these forces are applied during massage becomes the mode of application.

The historical terms used to describe these forces are effleurage, pétrissage, tapotement and so forth. These terms are gradually being replaced with the terms gliding, kneading, percussion and oscillation. When force is applied to the tissue through the mode of application, this is called loading. The various forces listed above are outlined in more detail below (also see Figs 7.4 and 7.5).

Tension loading (Fig. 7.4B)

- Tension forces (also called tensile force) occur when two ends of a structure are pulled apart from one another
- Tension force is created by methods such as traction, longitudinal stretching, and stroking with tissue drag
- Tissues elongate under tension loading with the intent of lengthening shortened tissues
- Tension loading is also effective in moving body fluids
- Tension force is used during massage with applications that drag, glide, lengthen and stretch tissue to elongate connective tissues and lengthen short muscles
- Gliding and stretching make the most use of tension loading
- The distinguishing characteristic of gliding strokes, is that they are applied horizontally in relation to the tissues, generating a tensile force
- When applying gliding strokes, light pressure remains on the skin
- Moderate pressure extends through the subcutaneous layer of the skin to reach muscle tissue but

not so deep as to compress the tissue against the underlying bony structure

- Moderate to heavy pressure that puts sufficient drag on the tissue mechanically affects the connective tissue and the proprioceptors (spindle cells and Golgi tendon organs) found in the muscle
- Heavy pressure produces a distinctive compressive force of the soft tissue against the underlying or adjacent bone
- Strokes that use moderate pressure from the fingers and toes towards the heart, following the muscle fiber direction, are excellent for mechanical and reflexive stimulation of blood flow, particularly venous return and lymphatics
- Light to moderate pressure with short, repetitive gliding following the patterns for the lymph vessels, is the basis for manual lymph drainage.

Note: The traditional term effleurage describes a gliding stroke.

Compression loading (Fig. 7.4A)

- Compressive forces occur when two structures are pressed together
- Compression moves down into the tissues, with varying depths of pressure adding bending and compressive forces
- Compressive force is a component of massage application that is described as depth of pressure
- The manipulations of compression usually penetrate the subcutaneous layer, whereas in the resting position they stay on the skin surface
- Excess compressive force will rupture or tear muscle tissue, causing bruising and connective tissue damage. This is a concern when pressure is applied to deeper layers of tissue
- To avoid tissue damage, the massage therapist must distribute the compressive force of massage over a broad contact area on the body. Therefore, the more compressive the force being used to either assess or treat the tissue, the broader the base of contact with the tissue should be, to prevent injury
- Compressive force is used therapeutically to affect circulation, nerve stimulation, and connective tissue pliability
- Compression is effective as a rhythmic pump-like method to facilitate fluid dynamics. Tissue will shorten and widen increasing the pressure within the tissue and affecting fluid flow
- Compression is an excellent method for enhancing circulation
- The pressure against the capillary beds changes the pressure inside the vessels and encourages fluid exchange

- Compression appropriately applied to arteries allows back pressure to build, and when the compression is released, it encourages increased arterial flow
- Much of the effect of compression results from pressing tissue against the underlying bone, causing it to spread
- Sustained compression will result in more pliable connective tissue structures and is effective in reducing tissue density and binding
- Compression loading is a main method of trigger point treatment.

Bending loading (Fig. 7.4C)

- Bending forces are a combination of compression and tension
- One side of a structure is exposed to compressive forces while the other side is exposed to tensile forces
- Bending occurs during many massage applications
- Pressure is applied to the tissue, or force is applied across the fiber or across the direction of the muscles, tendons or ligaments, and fascial sheaths
- Bending forces are excellent for direct stretching of tissue
- Bending force is very effective in increasing connective tissue pliability and affecting proprioceptors in the tendons and belly of the muscles
- A variation of the application of bending force is skin rolling
- Applying deep bending forces attempts to lift the muscular component away from the bone but skin rolling lifts only the skin from the underlying muscle layer
- It has a warming and softening effect on the superficial fascia, causes reflexive stimulation of the spinal nerves, and is an excellent assessment method for trigger points
- Areas of 'stuck' skin often suggest underlying problems (see Ch. 6).

Shear loading (Fig. 7.4D)

- Shear forces move tissue back and forth creating a combined pattern of compression and elongation of tissue
- Shearing is a sliding force
- The massage method called friction uses shear force to generate physiological change by increasing connective tissue pliability and to insure that tissue layers slide over one another instead of adhering to underlying layers, creating bind
- Application of friction also provides pain reduction through the mechanisms of counter-irritation and hyperstimulation analgesia (Yates 2004)

- Friction prevents and breaks up local adhesions in connective tissue, especially over tendons, ligaments and scars (Gehlsen et al 1999).

All of these outcomes of applying shear force during massage can address various factors influencing low back pain.

For example, hamstring muscles can adhere to each other or develop local areas of fibrosis from micro-trauma injury. The result is short, inflexible muscles that can be a contributing factor in low back dys-function. The lumbodorsal fascia can develop fibrotic areas that cause a decrease in pliability and a shortening of the structure, which can be a contributing factor in low back pain.

Trigger point referred pain patterns are aspects of back pain symptoms and the tissues surrounding trigger points that have been in place a long time may be fibrotic.

Friction is beneficial in these situations as properly applied shear force loading of the tissues can create a controlled inflammatory response that stimulates a change in tissue structure.

- Friction consists of small, deep movements performed on a local area
- The movement in friction is usually transverse to the fiber direction
- It is generally performed for 30 s to 10 min
- The result of this type of friction is initiation of a small, controlled inflammatory response
- The chemicals released during inflammation result in activation of tissue repair mechanisms together with reorganization of connective tissue
- As the tissue responds to the friction, the therapist should gradually begin to stretch the area and increase the pressure and intensity of the method
- The feeling for the client may be intense and typically described as burning, and if it is painful enough to produce flinching and guarding by the client, the application should be modified to a tolerable level so that the client reports the sensation as a 'good hurt'
- The recommended way to work within the client's comfort zone is to use pressure sufficient for him or her to feel the specific area, but not to feel the need to complain of pain
- The area being frictioned may be tender to the touch for 48 h after use of the technique
- The sensation should be similar to a mild after-exercise soreness
- Because the focus of friction is the controlled application of a small inflammatory response, heat and redness are caused by the release of histamine

- Also, increased circulation results in a small amount of puffiness as more water binds with the connective tissue
- The area should not bruise
- While using friction can be very beneficial there are cautions to applying excessive shear forces to tissues

Caution: This method is not used during an acute illness, or soon after an injury, or close to a fresh scar, and should only be used if adaptive capacity of the client can respond to superimposed tissue trauma.

- Excess friction (shearing force) may result in an inflammatory irritation that causes many soft tissue problems
- Friction will increase blood flow to an area but also cause edema from the resulting inflammation and tissue damage from the frictioning procedure
- The method is best used in small localized areas of connective tissue changes and to separate layers of tissue that might have become adhered
- The most common areas where more surface tissue becomes stuck to underlying structures are: scars, pectoralis major muscle adhering to pectoralis minor, rectus femoris adhering to vastus intero-medialis, gastrocnemius adhering to soleus, hamstring muscles adhering to each other, overlapping areas of tendons and ligaments.

Rotation or torsion loading (Fig. 7.4E)

- This force type is a combined application of compression and wringing, resulting in elongation of tissue along the axis of rotation
- It is used where a combined effect to both fluid dynamics and connective tissue pliability is desired
- Torsion forces are best thought of as twisting forces
- Massage methods that use kneading introduce torsion forces
- Soft tissue is lifted, rolled and squeezed
- Kneading soft tissue assesses changes in tissue texture and can be an aspect of treatment, especially as an aspect of stretching tissue or encouraging circulation or fluid movement in soft tissue
- Torsion force can be used therapeutically to affect connective tissue in the body
- Changes in depth of pressure and drag determine whether the kneading manipulation is perceived by the client as superficial or deep
- By the nature of the manipulation, the pressure and pull peak when the tissue is lifted to its maximum, and decrease at the beginning and end of the manipulation.

Note: pétrissage is another term for kneading.

Figure 7.4A–E Effects of mechanical forces produced during massage. (From Fritz S 2004 Fundamentals of therapeutic massage, 3rd edn. Mosby, St Louis.)

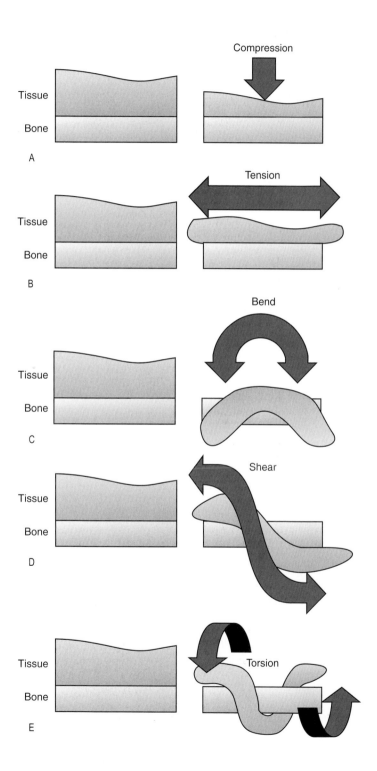

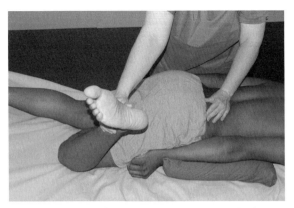

Figure 7.5 Combined loading example. Compression loading on soft tissue surrounding SI joint combined with passive joint movement creating tension loading. (Reproduced with kind permission from Mosby's Massage Career Development Series 2006.)

Combined loading

- Combining two or more forces effectively loads tissue (Fig. 7.5)
- The more forces applied to tissue the more intense the response
- Tension and compression underlie all the different modes of loading, therefore any form of manipulation is either tension, compression or a combination
- Tension is important in conditions where tissue needs to be elongated and compression where fluid flow needs to be affected.

JOINT MOVEMENT METHODS

- Joint movement is incorporated into massage for both assessment and treatment
- Joint movement is used to position muscles in preparation for muscle energy methods and before stretching tissues
- Joint movement also encourages fluid movement in the lymphatic, arterial and venous circulation systems
- Much of the pumping action that moves these fluids in the vessels results from rhythmic compression during joint movement and muscle contraction
- The tendons, ligaments, and joint capsules are warmed from joint movement
- This mechanical effect helps keep these tissues pliable.

Types of joint movement methods

Joint movement involves moving the jointed areas within the physiologic limits of range of motion of the

client. The two basic types of joint movement used during massage are active and passive.

Active joint movement means that the client moves the joint by active contraction of muscle groups. The two variations of active joint movement are as follows:

1 Active assisted movement, which occurs when both the client and the massage practitioner move the area
2 Active resistive movement, which occurs when the client actively moves the joint against a resistance provided by the massage practitioner.

Passive joint movement occurs when the client's muscles stay relaxed and the massage practitioner moves the joint with no assistance from the client. Various forms of oscillation (rocking and shaking) involve passive joint movement. Since muscle energy techniques are focused on specific muscles or muscle groups, it is important to be able to position muscles so that the muscle attachments are either close together or in a lengthening phase with the attachments separated.

- Joint movement is how this positioning is accomplished (Fig. 7.6)
- Joint movement is effective for positioning tissues to be stretched
- The muscles nearer the surface are relatively easy to position during the massage using joint movement
- The method can also be used for the smaller deeper joints of the spine and surrounding muscles but the positioning needs to be precise and focused
- Shortened tissue located in deep layers of muscle, or in a muscle that is difficult to lengthen by moving the body, can be addressed with local bending, shearing, and torsion in order to lengthen and stretch the local area, and this is easy to accomplish during the course of the massage.

Regardless of the massage methods practiced, or the massage style, the previous explanations: qualities of touch, mode of application to apply mechanical forces to affect the body in various mechanical and reflexive ways, in order to achieve specific outcomes, should create a generic base for communicating and understanding massage application.

MASSAGE APPLICATION FOR LOW BACK PAIN AND DYSFUNCTION

This section of the chapter provides suggestions and protocols (based on the author's experience) for using massage to address low back pain.

Information provided includes:

- general suggestions for massage for those with low back pain

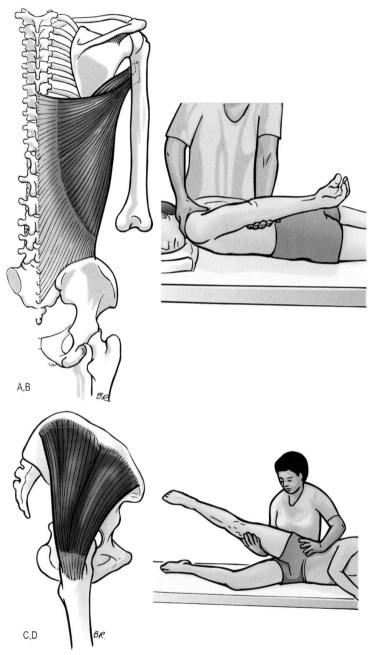

Figure 7.6 Examples of using joint movement to position muscles for treatment such as muscle energy techniques. (A,B) Latissimus dorsi, (C,D) gluteus medius.

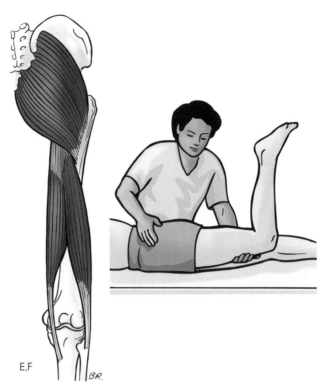

Figure 7.6, cont'd (E,F) gluteus maximus and hamstrings. (From Fritz S 2004 Fundamentals of therapeutic massage, 3rd edn. Mosby, St Louis.)

Box 7.1   Sequence of massage based on clinical reasoning to achieve specific outcomes

- Massage application intent (outcome) determines mode of application and variation on quality of touch:
  - *Mode of application*: influenced by type/mode of application (glide, knead, oscillation compression, percussion, movement, etc.)
  - *Quality of touch*: location of application, depth of pressure (light to deep), tissue drag, rate (speed) of application, rhythm, direction, frequency (number of repetitions) and duration of application of the method
- Mode of application with variations in quality of touch generate:
- Mechanical forces (tension, compression, bend, shear, torsion to affect tissue changes from physical loading) leading to:

- Influence on physiology
  - mechanical changes (tissue repair, connective tissue viscosity and pliability, fluid dynamic)
  - neurologic changes (stimulus response-motor system and neuromuscular, pain reflexes, mechanoreceptors)
  - psycho-physiologic changes (changes in mood, pain perception, sympathetic and parasympathetic balance)
- Interplay with unknown pathways and physiology (energetic, meridians, chakras, etc.)
  - contribute to development of treatment approach
  - resulting in desired outcomes.

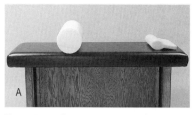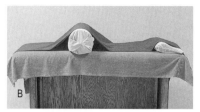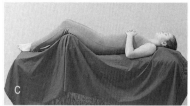

Figure 7.7   Supine positioning. (From Fritz S 2004 Fundamentals of therapeutic massage, 3rd edn. Mosby/Elsevier, St Louis).

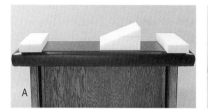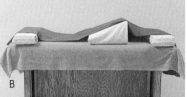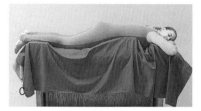

Figure 7.8   Prone positioning. (From Fritz S 2004 Fundamentals of therapeutic massage, 3rd edn. Mosby, St Louis.)

- massage strategies for back pain, connective tissue dysfunction and breathing dysfunction
- strategies for specific muscles involved in low back pain
- strategies for joints involved in low back pain
- massage treatment for acute back pain
- massage protocol for common low back conditions.

General suggestions for using massage to treat low back pain

- When the person is supine (Fig. 7.7), make sure the knees are flexed slightly and bolstered so that strain is taken off the low back.
- Do not keep the person with low back pain in the prone position (Fig. 7.8) for too long since this stresses the back musculature
- Use side-lying position with bolstering
- When the person is prone, place a pillow under their abdomen so the spine is in a more normal position
- The surface muscles of the low back region are typically larger and thicker than the muscles in other body areas. This makes reaching the deeper soft tissue structures more difficult. It is necessary to systematically work through the muscle layers and maintain a broad based contact on the surface tissues as increasing pressure is applied to reach the more problematic deeper structures
- The postural muscles and the surface phasic muscles of the low back region often increase in motor tone to stabilize instability in the joints. This is resourceful compensation. Do not over-work the area by expecting complete relief after the massage.

More realistic goals are a 50% reduction in pain and increased mobility with the remaining sensations interpreted as stiffness rather than pain
- Trigger point activity in the belly of muscles is usually located in short concentrically contracted muscles
- These are the trigger points to be targeted during the massage if they relate to the low back pain
- Trigger points located near the attachments are usually found in eccentric patterns in long inhibited muscles acting as antagonists to concentrically contracted muscles and it is usually best to leave these trigger points alone
- Do not overtreat in any one session
- Only address the soft tissue dysfunctions that recreate the symptoms the client is experiencing; this is especially true of the specific muscle releases and trigger points
- Remember anything can feel like a trigger point or a painful muscle if pressed on hard enough
- Only address the trigger points that are most painful, most medial and most proximal and that recreate the client's low back symptoms
- Leave the rest alone and monitor them over the course of three or four massage sessions to identify improvement
- When the posture and function normalize with regular massage, the trigger point activity will often resolve
- When performing the specific muscle releases, choose one or two muscles to address during the massage session and then monitor the results

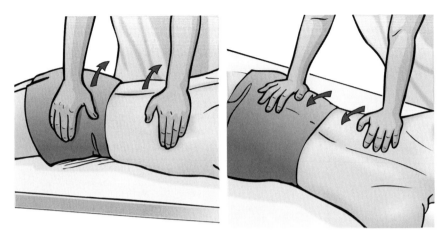

Figure 7.9   Example of rocking the lumbar area. (From Fritz S 2004 Fundamentals of therapeutic massage, 3rd edn. Mosby, St Louis.)

- It is best to address the low back issues in the short tissues first, and wait to see if the soft tissue dysfunctions in 'lengthened muscles', and at the attachments, resolve, as the posture of muscle interaction normalizes
- Both the massage methods and the joint movements (active and passive) used during massage should be applied in a slow, deliberate manner
- Sudden, quick movements can lead to spasm and are likely to increase muscle tension by over stimulating the nerve receptors
- Oscillation movements, such as shaking and rocking, are very effective in reducing motor tone in hyperreactive muscles, especially those that are guarding. Unfortunately, most of the muscles responsible for low back pain are not easily shaken and so sustained rhythmic rocking of the whole body may be effective
- During the massage, intermittently gently rock the person for 1–2 min, then return to the massage strokes (Fig. 7.9)
- Expect that it will take a series of 12 massage sessions before sustainable improvement is noticed
- If the client feels very loose after the massage and is much worse the next day, the massage may have destabilized adaptive compensating mechanisms in the low back area. The work was probably too aggressive, resulting in a reflexive increase in the guarding response. The client should improve over the next 3–4 days. Reduce the intensity of the massage and target general relaxation responses.

MASSAGE STRATEGIES FOR BACK PAIN

Generalized pain management

Massage application targeted to low back pain management incorporates the following principles:

1   General full-body application with a rhythmic and slow approach, as often as feasible with 45–60 min durations. *Goal*: Parasympathetic dominance with reduced cortisol.
2   Pressure depth is moderate to deep with compressive broad-based application. No poking, frictioning, or application of pain-causing methods. *Goal*: Serotonin and GABA support and reduce substance P and adrenaline.
3   Drag is slight unless connective tissue is being targeted. Drag is targeted to lymphatic drain and skin stimulation. Massage for simple back pain is best combined with hot and cold hydrotherapy, and counterirritant ointment. *Goal*: Reduce swelling and create counterirritation through skin stimulation.
4   Nodal points on the body that have a high neurovascular component are massaged with a sufficient depth of pressure to create a 'good hurt' sensation but not defensive guarding or withdrawal. These nodal points are the location of cutaneous nerves, trigger points, acupuncture points, reflexology points, etc. The foot, hands and head, as well as along the spine, are excellent target locations. *Goal*: Gate control response, endorphin and other pain-inhibiting chemical release.

Figure 7.10   Using tension force to hold tissue at bind. (From Fritz S 2004 Fundamentals of therapeutic massage, 3rd edn. Mosby, St Louis.)

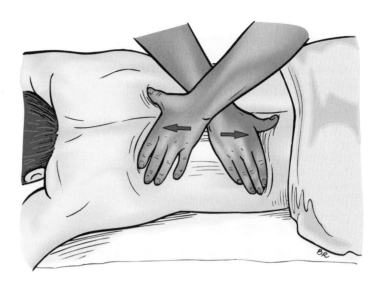

5   Direction of massage varies, but deliberately targets fluid movement. *Goal*: Circulation.

6   Mechanical force introduction of shear, bend, torsion, etc., are of an agitation quality to 'stir' the ground substance and not create inflammation. *Goal*: Increased tissue pliability and reduced tissue density.

7   Mechanical force application of shear, bend and torsion is used to address adhesion or fibrosis but needs to be specifically targeted and limited in duration. *Goal*: Reduced localized nerve irritation or circulation reduction.

8   Muscle energy methods and lengthening are applied rhythmically, gently, and targeted to shortened muscles. *Goal*: Reduced nerve and proprioceptive irritation and circulation inhibition.

9   Stretching to introduce tension force is applied slowly, without pain and targeted to shortened connective tissue. *Goal*: Reduce nerve and proprioceptive irritation.

10   Massage therapists are focused, attentive, compassionate, but maintain appropriate boundaries. *Goal*: Support entrainment, bioenergy normalization and palliative care.

Additional methods that modulate pain sensation and perception that can be incorporated into the massage are: simple applications of hot and cold hydrotherapy, analgesic essential oils, calming and distracting music.

Connective tissue approaches

Changes in the connective tissue structures in the low back area are often identified as short or thick during assessment. The lumbo-dorsal fascial, iliotibial band and associated fascia of the thigh, and fascial structures of the anterior thorax are typically involved. Increasing pliability in these structures seems to reduce the symptoms of stiffness. Be cautious in how intensely the connective tissue is massaged, since the shortening may be an aspect of increased stability in the area.

The important consideration for connective tissue massage methods is that the pressure vertically and horizontally actually moves the tissue to create tension, torsion, shear or bend forces, which triggers alteration of the ground substance long enough for energy to build up in it and soften it. The development of connective tissue patterns is highly individualized, and because of this, systems that follow a precise protocol and sequence are often less effective in dealing with these complex patterns.

A good grip with the skin is essential, so there must be no lotion or oil present. This grip can be with the hands or forearms. The technique is sometimes performed without a towel, to provide stronger contact with the skin.

Tissues can be moved towards 'ease' (the way they want to move) and the position is held for a few seconds to allow the tissues to soften. The client can move the tissues by contracting or relaxing the muscle as the massage therapist holds the tissue at ease. The entire procedure can be repeated holding the tissues at 'bind' (the way they do not want to move) (Fig. 7.10).

Tissue movement methods

The more subtle connective tissue approaches rely on the skilled development of following tissue movement. The process is as follows:

- Make firm but gentle contact with the skin
- Increase the downward, or vertical, pressure slowly until resistance is felt; this barrier is soft and subtle
- Maintain the downward pressure at this point; now add horizontal pressure until the resistance barrier is felt again
- Sustain the horizontal pressure and wait
- The tissue will seem to creep, unravel, melt, slide, quiver, twist, or dip, or some other movement sensation will be apparent
- Follow the movement, gently maintaining the tension on the tissue, encouraging the pattern as it undulates though various levels of release
- Slowly and gently release first the horizontal force and then the vertical force.

Twist-and-release kneading and compression applied in the direction of the restriction can also release these fascial barriers.

BREATHING DYSFUNCTION

As described in Chapter 4, dysfunctional breathing is a common aspect of back pain.

The massage therapist influences breathing in two distinct ways:

1 Supporting balance between sympathetic and parasympathetic autonomic nervous systems function. This is generally accomplished with a relaxation focus to the general full body massage.
2 Normalizing and then maintaining effective thoracic and respiratory muscle function.

The following protocol specifically targets these areas. The applications would be integrated into the general massage protocol to work more specifically with breathing function if assessment indicates any tendency to breathing pattern dysfunction. It is strongly recommended that the reader studies the textbook *Multidisciplinary Approaches to Breathing Pattern Disorders* (Chaitow et al 2002).

Assessment

Observe and palpate for overuse of upper chest breathing muscles during normal relaxed breathing using the information in Chapter 4.

In addition, the following assessments are easily incorporated into the massage:

- The massage therapist stands behind the seated client and places his or her hands over the upper trapezius area so that the tips of the fingers rest on the top of the clavicles
- As the client breathes, determine if the accessory muscles are being used for relaxed breathing. If the shoulders move up and down as the client breathes,

it is likely that accessory muscles are being recruited. In normal relaxed breathing, the shoulders should not move in this way. The client will be using accessory muscles to breathe if the chest movement is concentrated in the upper chest instead of the lower ribs and abdomen

- Using any of the accessory muscles for breathing results in an increase in tension and tendency towards the development of trigger points. These situations can be identified with palpation. Connective tissue changes are common, since this breathing dysfunction is often chronic. The connective tissues are palpated as thick, dense and shortened in this area
- Have the client inhale and exhale, and observe for a consistent exhalation that is longer than the inhalation. Normal relaxed breathing consists of a shorter inhalation phase in relationship to a longer exhalation phase. The ratio of inhalation time to exhalation is one count inhalation to four counts exhalation. A reverse of this pattern indicates a breathing pattern disorder. The ideal pattern would range between 2–4 counts during the inhalation and 8–10 counts for the exhalation. Targeted massage and breathing retraining methods can be used to restore normal relaxed breathing
- Have the client hold their breath without strain to assess for tolerance to carbon dioxide levels. They should be able to comfortably hold the breath for at least 15 s, with 30 s being ideal
- Palpate and gently mobilize the thorax to assess for rib mobility. This is done in supine, prone, sidelying and seated positions. The ribs should have a springy feel, and be a bit more mobile from the 6th to the 10th ribs.

Treatment

The following muscles are specifically targeted by massage because they tend to shorten during breathing dysfunction:

- scalenes
- sternocleidomastoid
- serratus anterior
- serratus posterior superior and inferior
- levator scapulae
- rhomboids
- upper trapezius
- pectoralis major and minor
- latissimus dorsi
- psoas
- quadratus lumborum
- all abdominals
- calf muscles.

The intercostals and diaphragm, which are the main breathing muscles, should also be addressed.

- All of these muscles should be assessed for shortening, weakness and agonist/antagonist interaction. Muscles that orient mostly transverse, such as the serratus anterior, serratus posterior superior and inferior, rhomboids and pelvic floor muscles, are difficult to assess with movement and strength testing. Palpation (see Ch. 6) will be more accurate. The typical patterns of the upper and lower crossed syndromes are often involved
- Muscles assessed as short need to be lengthened. If the primary cause of the shortening is neuro-muscular, then use inhibitory pressure at the muscle belly and lengthen either by moving the adjacent joints, or more likely, by introducing tension, bend or torsion force directly on the muscle tissues
- For the scalenes, sternocleidomastoid, serratus anterior, pectoralis minor, latissimus dorsi, psoas, quadratus lumborum, diaphragm, rectus abdominis and pelvic floor muscles, follow recommendations about specific release methods later in this chapter
- Work with each area as needed, as it becomes convenient during the general massage session. Use the least invasive measure possible to restore a more normal muscle resting length
- If the breathing has been dysfunctional for an extended period of time (over 3 months) connective tissue changes are common. Focused connective tissue massage application is effective
- Once the soft tissue is more normal, then gentle mobilization of the thorax is appropriate. If the thoracic vertebrae and ribs are restricted, chiro-practic or other joint manipulation methods may be appropriate and referral is indicated. The massage therapist can use indirect functional techniques to increase the mobility of the area as well. These methods are described in general in Chapter 6.

Methods and sequence used to address the breathing function need to be integrated into a full body approach, since breathing is a whole body function. A possible protocol to add to the general massage session would be as follows:

- Increased attention to general massage of the thorax; posterior, anterior and lateral access to the thorax is used primarily to address the general tension or dysfunctional patterns in the respiratory muscles of this area
- Address the scalenes, psoas and quadratus lumborum and legs, especially calves
- Use appropriate muscle energy techniques to lengthen and stretch the shortened muscles of the cervical, thoracic, and lumbar regions and legs

- Gently move the rib cage with broad-based compression
- Assess for areas that move easily and those that are restricted
- Assess the anterior, lateral and posterior areas
- Identify the amount of rigidity in the ribs with the client supine by applying bilateral compression to the thorax beginning near the clavicles and moving down towards the lower ribs maintaining compressive force near the costal cartilage
- Identify rigidity in the ribs with the client prone bilaterally (on both sides of the spine) at the facet joints beginning near the 7th cervical vertebra and moving down towards the lower ribs maintaining compressive force near the facet joints
- The breathing wave assessment can also confirm areas of restriction (see p. 51, Fig. 4.13)
- Compression against the lateral aspect of the thorax with the client in a side-lying position will assess rib mobility in both facet and costal joints
- Begin applying the compression near the axilla and then moving down towards the lower ribs
- Sufficient force needs to be used while applying the compression to feel the ribs spring but not so much as to cause discomfort
- Normal response would be a feeling of equal mobility bilaterally
- A feeling of stiffness or rigidity would indicate immobility
- Identify the area of most mobility and the area of most restriction
- Position the client so that a broad-based compressive force can be applied to the areas of ease – the most mobile
- Gently and slowly apply compression until the area begins to bind
- Hold this position and have the client cough
- Coughing will act as a muscle energy method and also support mobility of the joint through activation of the muscles
- Repeat three or four times.

If areas of rigidity remain, the following intervention may be useful:

- Apply broad-based compression to the area of immobility (Fig. 7.11) using the whole hand or forearm
- Have the client exhale, then increase the intensity of the compressive force while following the exhalation
- Hold the ribs in this position
- Have the client push out against the compressive pressure
- Instruct the client to inhale while continuing to hold the compressive focus against the ribs

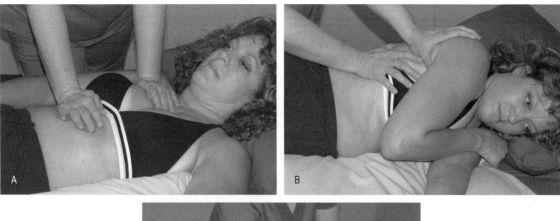

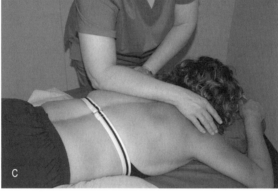

Figure 7.11   Examples of broad based compression to the ribs. (Reproduced with kind permission from Mosby's Massage Career Development Series 2006.)

- Then have the client exhale while following the action of the ribs. There should be an increase in mobility
- Gently mobilize the entire thorax with rhythmic compression. Reassess the area of most bind/restriction. If the areas treated have improved, then a different area is located and the sequence is repeated. It is appropriate to do three or four areas in a session
- Palpate for tender points in the intercostals, pectoralis minor and anterior serratus (clients are not very tolerant of this so be directive and precise).

Use positional release to release these points by moving the client or having them move into various positions until the pain in the tender point decreases. The procedure for positional release is as follows:

- Locate the tender point
- Gently initiate the pain response with direct pressure (remember the sensation of pain is a guide only)
- The pain point is not the point of intervention

- Slowly position the body, actively or passively, until the pain subsides. This position can be focal and accomplished by moving the client's ribs, arm or head, or a whole body process involving many different areas to achieve the position where there is a decrease in the pain
- Maintain the position for up to 30 s or until the client feels the release, while encouraging them to breathe from the diaphragm, lightly monitoring the tender point
- Slowly reposition the client to neutral and then into a stretch position for the tender point
- Direct tissue stretching is usually most effective.

If the client is sniffling, coughing, sneezing, or has been laughing a lot, then the posterior serratus inferior can be the cause of back pain. This muscle tends to shorten due to its stabilizing function of the lower ribs.

- Because of its fiber direction, it is very difficult to stretch
- The symptoms include an aching sensation just below the scapula at the location of the muscle

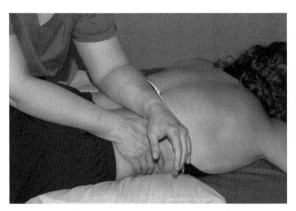

Figure 7.12 Compression on posterior serratus inferior. (Reproduced with kind permission from Mosby's Massage Career Development Series 2006.)

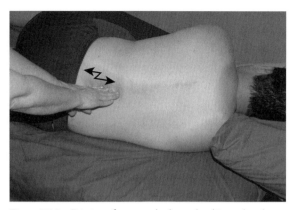

Figure 7.13 Friction of paravertebral muscles. (Reproduced with kind permission from Mosby's Massage Career Development Series 2006.)

- Compression into the muscle belly (Fig. 7.12) with local tissue stretching usually relieves the symptoms.

Once the thorax and breathing function begins to normalize – usually after 4–6 focused sessions – then it is appropriate to teach a simple breathing exercise. Often massage focused to normalized breathing is sufficient to address most causal factors in low back pain.

STRATEGIES FOR SPECIFIC MUSCLES INVOLVED IN LOW BACK PAIN

Muscle firing pattern dysfunction is almost always present and is discussed in Chapter 5. Assessment and treatment should be included in massage and suggestions will be provided later in the sample protocol.

Massage should be targeted at the following muscles: paravertebral muscles, psoas, quadratus lumborum, groin muscle attachment, hamstrings, and gluteal group including deep lateral rotations.

Specific assessment and release methods for these muscles that are easily incorporated into massage are described below. The intervention used to normalize muscle motor tone and length is inhibitory pressure in the belly of the muscle if possible and occasionally at the attachments if access to the muscle belly is difficult. The client is positioned so the compression applied to the muscle is effective.

Paravertebral muscles

Multifidi, rotators, intertransversarii and interspinalis: as a combined group, these muscles produce small refined movements of the vertebral column. They work in coordination, with each small group of muscle fibers contributing to the entire action.

Symptoms
- Clients often feel as though they want to have their back 'cracked' yet manipulation does not necessarily provide relief
- There is stiffness upon initiation of movement but once the movement begins, the stiffness is reduced
- The client is unable to stretch effectively to affect these muscle groups
- The client experiences an aching as opposed to a sharp pain.

Assessment
Palpation is an effective assessment. These are small deep muscles basically located between the vertebrae. A history of sitting or fixed standing for extended periods of time is common. Palpation, with the client both prone and side-lying, deep into the spaces between the vertebrae will reveal tough tissue bands that may replicate the symptoms. Effective palpation must go deep enough to contact the muscle group and get under the erector spinae muscles.

Procedures
- Meticulous frictioning of the tight muscle bands combined with tissue stretching (Fig. 7.13)
- Softening and lengthening the erector spine and associated fascia are necessary before beginning the methods
- Position the client in the side-lying position with the affected side up and with a small amount of passive extension

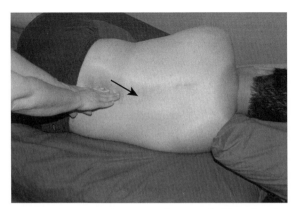

Figure 7.14   Position for massage of paraspinals. (Reproduced with kind permission from Mosby's Massage Career Development Series 2006.)

- Angle in at 45° against the groove next to the spinal column using braced double fingers or a massage tool (Fig. 7.14)
- Sink in until you can feel the spinous processes
- Hold the compression firmly against the affected tissue and have the client slowly move the area back and forth from extension to flexion. This movement is very small and focused and is performed in a rocking fashion
- Then have the client remain in a slight extension while you move your fingers down in a deep scooping action and then out again, as if you were digging or scooping
- After the tissue has softened further, firmly hold the compression and have the client move into spinal flexion very slowly until you feel the tissue become taut, in order to stretch the area
- Hold this position until the tissue softens.

Psoas

Symptoms
- Client complains of generalized lumbar aching
- Aching into top of the thighs
- Low back pain when coughing, sneezing
- Pain when lying on the stomach
- Pain when lying flat on back.

Assessment
- Gait stride shortened, more so on the short side
- Externally rotated leg on the short side
- Bracing with hands when sitting down or standing up
- Leg unable to fall into full extension, as shown in the supine edge of table test below (see Positioning)
- Anteriorly tipped pelvis.

Note: A tight and/or shortened quadratus group and tensor fasciae latae are often found together with psoas dysfunction, and should be addressed before dealing with the psoas muscles.

End of table psoas test   This test is done by having the client place their ischial tuberosities on the edge of the table, bringing one leg to the chest and rolling back to lie on the table. When the leg is held tightly to the chest the other leg should lie horizontally, parallel with the table. If the thigh is angled upward from the table, psoas on that side is short.

Sit-up test   Client lies supine on the table with the knees bent. Arms are extended and slightly angled towards the ceiling ('sleep walking position').
- The client then lifts his/her torso off the table by reaching for the ceiling
- The practitioner holds or observes both feet
- The foot on the side of a short psoas will lift off the table first.

Procedures
Muscle energy lengthening and stretch in all positions: edge of table, side-lying, supine edge of table, over side of table and prone.

Positioning (Fig. 7.15)
1 *Supine edge of table*: Make sure pelvis is fixed firmly to the table and the knee on the opposite side is rolled as close to the chest as possible. Hand placement for resistance force and lengthening is above the knee.
2 *Supine*: Client lies close to the edge of the table and bends the knee not near the edge. The psoas being addressed is accessed by having the client drop the leg over the edge of the table to achieve lengthening and stretching. The pelvis must be fixed and stabilized.
3 *Side-lying*: Bottom leg is drawn up towards the chest and the practitioner is positioned behind the client. The torso remains fixed and the lumbar area is stabilized. The client bends the top knee and the practitioner cradles the thigh in her arm. The top leg is then slightly internally rotated, abducted and extended.
4 *Prone*: Pelvis is fixed to the table. The practitioner is positioned opposite the side to be addressed. The leg remains straight on the side closest to the practitioner. The knee of the target leg is flexed past 90° and the hip slightly internally rotated (accomplished by allowing the foot to fall a bit to the outside) to prepare that side to be lengthened and stretched. The practitioner reaches across and cradles the anterior thigh in her arm, lifts up and leans back.

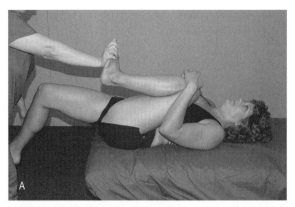
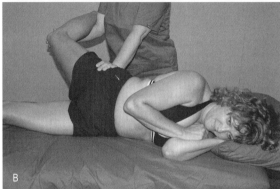
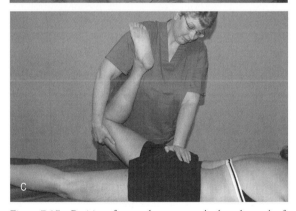

Figure 7.15   Positions for muscle energy methods and stretch of the psoas (A) supine (B) side-lying (C) prone. (Reproduced with kind permission from Mosby's Massage Career Development Series 2006.)

Note: Decisions on which of these four positions is the most effective will depend on the reports of the client and the size of the client in relation to the practitioner.

Direct access of psoas using hand and/or fist
The psoas muscle can be accessed in either the supine or side-lying position, whichever is most effective.

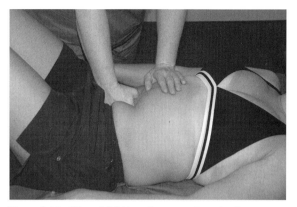

Figure 7.16   Direct inhibition of psoas supine using fist. (Reproduced with kind permission from Mosby's Massage Career Development Series 2006.)

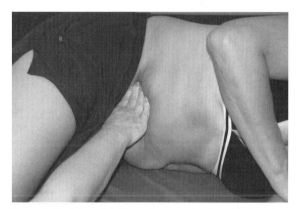

Figure 7.17   Direct inhibition of psoas side-lying using braced hand. (Reproduced with kind permission from Mosby's Massage Career Development Series 2006.)

- Client is supine with the knees flexed to at least 110°
- Both feet are flat on the table
- The practitioner stands on the side to be addressed
- Either a flat stabilized hand or a loose fist can be used
- Decision is based on the size and comfort of the client
- For the practitioner, the fist position will withstand a longer duration of treatment (Fig. 7.16)
- With client side-lying and knees flexed, the practitioner kneels in front of the client and leans in using a stabilized hand or loose fist (Fig. 7.17)
- The leg can be used to pull the client towards the pressure

- The muscle location is best accessed midline between the iliac crest and the navel and can usually be found by placing the metacarpophalangeal joint on the iliac crest
- The fingers remain straight and the tip of the fingers identifies the location of the muscle
- This muscle is located deep against the anterior aspect of the lumbar and lower thoracic spine
- Slow deliberate compression into the lower abdomen is required
- The ovary is tucked under the ilea and must not be compressed
- The abdominal aorta can be palpated as pulsation and must not be compressed
- The small and large intestine will slide out of the way with an undulating action as the downward and angled force towards the spine is exerted
- Identification of the proper location can be confirmed by having the client flex the leg which would activate the psoas
- A flat sustained compression is used in conjunction with having the client slowly move the head and neck into flexion, side flexion and rotation in all directions in order to facilitate the psoas and act to contract/then relax the muscle while pressure is maintained
- The psoas can also be inhibited by having the client activate the neck extensor by slightly tipping the chin towards the ceiling and pushing the back of the head against the table
- Alternating flexion and extension of the neck is valuable while maintaining inhibitory pressure against the psoas
- All these neck actions can be supplemented with eye movement: eyes look downward during forward flexion, sideways during lateral flexion and upward during extension
- Additionally, the client can slowly slide the heel of the foot out so that the leg becomes straight
- When the leg is straight, if the client contracts the buttock muscles, the psoas is further inhibited
- Then the client relaxes the gluteal muscles and draws the heel as close to the buttocks as possible to contract the psoas
- This action is repeated while the compression on the psoas is maintained.

Release at the distal attachment:

- If it is difficult to access the psoas through the abdomen then inhibiting pressure near the distal attachment where the muscle crosses the pubic bone is possible. Usually the leg is moved into an ease or bind position, while the inhibiting pressure is held

- The compression of the psoas acts to lengthen and stretch this muscle.

After this treatment, make sure the client does not get right off the table, but instead rolls first to the side and then rolls up. Assist if necessary. Do not let the client sit straight up.

- Having the client lay prone is a gentle lengthening position for this muscle
- Then have the client assume a four-point position by getting on to hands and knees in order to perform the cat or sway back position and camel or hunch back position
- Then have the client slide his/her arms in front while bringing the buttocks back against the hamstrings
- Apply broad based compression against the lumbar area in this position
- If the psoas is not acute, then have the client drop gently into the cobra position by lifting the head and chest, straightening the arms, and placing the pelvis flat against the table
- Each position is held up to 3 min based on what feels good
- The client then assumes the hands and knees position to get off the table.

All methods described can be used in coordination for a more intense interaction. The goal is to reduce tension in the psoas muscles. This is usually palpated as a sinking-in, or a feeling of 'giving' of the tissues. The client will usually modify the breathing pattern by taking a deep breath and relaxing when the muscle lets go.

This is a painful and intense procedure. Give the client breaks during the procedure by decreasing the pressure a bit but do not lose contact with the muscle since it is uncomfortable to relocate it. Expect the muscle to relax in 30 s.

If no change is identified in 60 s, it is likely that the muscle will not respond to treatment during that session.

Rehabilitation exercises (see Ch. 8)

Quadratus lumborum

Symptoms
- Deep local low back pain which may be more on one side
- Pain radiation into buttocks and down the side of the leg to the knee (nerve entrapment)
- Tends to wiggle or attempts to stretch with lateral trunk flexion
- May have restricted breathing
- Short leg on affected side (may be functional or physical).

Assessment

- Position client on their side. Palpate with either the forearms or hands in the space between the ribs and the iliac crest. Have the client straighten and then lift the top leg. The area being palpated should not activate until the leg is raised above 20°. If it does, the quadratus is tense and short
- Have the client lie prone with legs straight and assess leg length. The short leg may indicate a tight quadratus lumborum. If lateral flexion of the torso is restricted or asymmetrical, the most restriction will be on the side away from which lateral flexion is taking place.

Procedures

- Position client on side with bottom leg bent and top leg straight and in slight hip extension
- While standing behind the client, apply compression into the space between the last rib and the top of the iliac crest
- The angle of force is about 70° (angled towards the navel)
- When resistance is felt in the muscle, have the client lift the top leg up and down
- Make sure the hip stays in extension
- Have the client alternately move the neck and head back and forth in lateral flexion and extension
- Both of these moves facilitate or inhibit the quadratus lumborum muscles
- These neck movements can be supplemented with side-to-side eye movements
- After the muscle releases it will need to be lengthened and stretched
- Stabilize the thorax and lengthen by dropping the top leg even more into a lengthened and stretched position
- Use a manual stretch by alternately exerting a force into the low back towards the navel and side-bending the client in extension, with both the torso and the leg
- Self-help could include: fingers interlaced, palms turned up and arms extended over the head. The pelvis is held stable and rolled forward either standing, or on knees. Side bend and twist into slight flexion. Perform the stretch on both sides with more emphasis on the affected quadratus lumborum (Fig. 7.18).

Deep lateral hip rotators

Symptoms

- Externally rotated foot
- Pain deep in gluteal region, which may be in conjunction with impinged sciatic nerve.

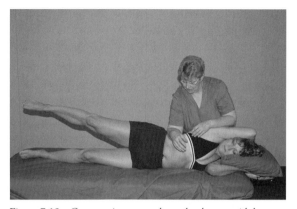

Figure 7.18   Compression on quadratus lumborum with leg movement. (Reproduced with kind permission from Mosby's Massage Career Development Series 2006.)

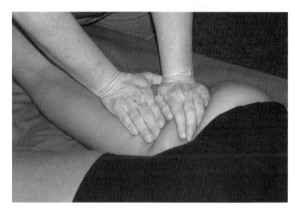

Figure 7.19   Compression with movement on deep lateral hip rotators. (Reproduced with kind permission from Mosby's Massage Career Development Series 2006.)

Assessment

- Physical assessment for externally rotated foot
- Palpation into the belly of the muscle to identify tender points that recreate symptoms.

Procedures

Compression with internal and external rotation of deep lateral rotators.

Stretching

While in the prone position:

- Lean into upper gluteal area on the target side, delivering pressure by using fist or forearm (Fig. 7.19)
- Without extending the hip on the target side, passively flex the knee to 90° by using your other hand to lift ankle

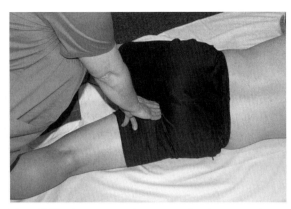

Figure 7.20   Assessment and treatment of groin area muscles. (Reproduced with kind permission from Mosby's Massage Career Development Series 2006.)

- When you move that lower leg medially so the ankle is behind the knee of the other leg, this places muscles in passive contraction (lateral rotation of hip)
- If you are leaning on the correct gluteal spot, the client's contracting muscles will push back against your pressure
- Change position of your pressure until this passive contraction does push back. Then perform an opposite lateral motion of the lower leg (medial rotation of hip), which places muscles into passive stretch
- You can use tense and relax, reciprocal inhibition, contract-relax-antagonist-contract, or pulsed muscle energy to accomplish release
- While in the supine position, the muscles can be stretched
- Due to the placement of attachments, in the supine position with the hip flexed to 90° the leg is externally rotated and pulled towards the chest.

Groin area muscles

Symptoms
- Sensation of high groin pull, but not able to palpate tenderness in the adductor region
- Restricted breathing
- Shortened stride.

Assessment
- Assess by palpation (Fig. 7.20)
- Have client lie on side with top leg bent and pulled up
- Using the supported hand position with flat fingers, contact the ischial tuberosity from the

inferior approach on the bottom and slide over it with a downward 45° angle, moving superiorly and medially on the client's body
- Shift direction of force to identify tender areas that recreate symptoms.

Procedures
- Maintain contact with the tender points that create symptoms, increase compressive force and have the client slightly extend and gently adduct bottom leg
- Continue pressure until you feel the muscle give way and let you in deeper
- Be sure to perform this procedure on both right and left sides, or the client will feel unbalanced when walking.

MASSAGE STRATEGIES FOR JOINTS RELATED TO LOW BACK PAIN

Sacroiliac (SI) joint dysfunction is a major cause of pain that requires a multidisciplinary approach (see Ch. 5). The joint can be jammed, unstable or fused, which interferes with pelvic function and movement during gait. The restricted pelvic movement creates increased movement at L4–5, S-I area or to the hip, or both. Pain commonly occurs in the hip abductors and around the coccyx/sacrum area on the affected side. Proper mobilization of the joint by an appropriate professional may be necessary. Massage supports the mobilization process by reducing muscle guarding and increasing tissue pliability. Once the joint is adjusted, the mobilization sequence for the SI joint can be incorporated into the general massage.

- The latissimus dorsi muscle opposite the symptomatic SI joint is part of the force couple that stabilizes the SI joint. The lumbo-dorsal fascia needs to be pliable but not so loose that stability is affected
- Commonly, the symphysis pubis is somewhat distressed in conjunction with SI joint dysfunction. A simple resistance method can address this condition. The client is supine, the knees are bent, and the massage therapist provides resistance against the action of the client's attempt to pull the knees together
- Apply a resistance force against the medial aspect of both knees. This can be done by holding the knees apart or placing the hand against one knee and the flat of the elbow against the other as the client attempts to pull their knees together
- The action activates the adductors and this may pull the symphysis pubis into a better alignment. Sometimes there is a 'popping' sound when the symphysis resets but that is not essential for effective results.

Often the sacrotuberous and sacrospinous ligaments are short, or the hamstring and gluteus maximus attachments near these ligaments are binding.

- Assess by palpation
- Have client lie on one side with the top leg bent and pulled up
- Using the supported hand, position with flat fingers, contact the ischial tuberosity from the inferior approach on the bottom (similar to position for groin muscle attachments)
- Shift direction of force to identify tender areas that recreate symptoms
- These ligament structures are difficult to reach, and when located, a compressive force is applied to the ligament while the client activates the hamstrings and gluteus maximus
- The results should be increased pliability of the ligament releasing the muscles to move more freely without bind.

If there is a functional long leg, the SI joint can become jammed on the long leg side.

- Typically the pelvis is anteriorly rotated on the symptomatic affected side and posteriorly rotated on the non-symptomatic side with quadratus lumborum short on the non-symptomatic side
- An indirect functional technique for anterior rotation, combined with quadratus lumborum release is often effective. The physical therapist (PT) or chiropractor rotates the pelvis and the massage therapist applies methods to normalize the soft tissue compensation. Firing patterns need to be assessed and normalized.

Sacroiliac (SI) joint and pelvis alignment (see p. 69)

The following describes assessment and treatment of back pain related to SI joint and pelvis issues, which can easily be incorporated into massage (Fig. 7.21).

Symptoms
- Pain over SI joint
- Increased symptoms when standing on one leg or when sleeping at night

Assessment
- With the client prone, apply direct compression over SI joint to identify if symptoms increase.

Treatment
- Stabilize the sacrum with the hand, foot or leg
- Have the prone client extend the hips alternately as if they were walking backwards

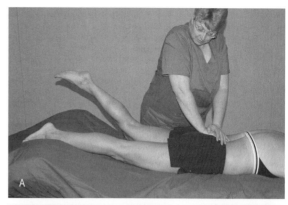

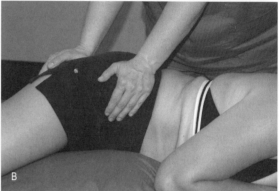

Figure 7.21   SI joint mobilization. (A) Stabilize sacrum and alternately extend thigh. (B) Compression to mobilize SI joint in multiple direction. (Reproduced with kind permission from Mosby's Massage Career Development Series 2006.)

- Next, move the joint by applying compression down (towards the table) alternately at the iliac crest and ischial tuberosity
- While the client is side-lying, compress the SI joint up and down, back and forth.

Indirect functional technique for the pelvis

First, assess for asymmetry by comparing both anterior superior iliac spines (ASIS) while the client is in the supine position.
   Dysfunction includes:

- Bilateral anterior rotation: ASIS palpates as forward and low
- Bilateral posterior rotation: ASIS palpates as backward and high
- Right or left anterior rotation: ASIS palpates as one low and one high
- Right or left posterior rotation: ASIS palpates as one low and one high
- Inflare is left, right or bilateral: ASIS angled towards midline

- Outflare left or right or bilateral: ASIS angled away from midline.

To correct using indirect functional technique: client is supine.

Anterior rotation
- Use leg to rotate pelvis into increased anterior rotation by bringing leg over edge of table
- Have client pull leg towards shoulder
- Apply moderate resistance and repeat three or four times
- Then on the final move, with the patient fully relaxed, ease the pelvis posteriorly by taking the knee towards the shoulder, without undue force, increasing posterior rotation.

Posterior rotation
- Begin with leg bent towards the shoulder increasing posterior rotation
- Have client push leg out and down over the table
- Apply moderate resistance and repeat three or four times
- Then on the final move, with the patient fully relaxed, ease the pelvis anteriorly by taking the knee towards the floor without undue force, increasing anterior rotation.

Inflare
- Position hip in flexion and internal rotation, increasing inflare
- Have client push out against moderate resistance
- Result is external rotation of hip
- Repeat three or four times
- Then on the final move, with the patient fully relaxed, ease the pelvis laterally by taking the knee away from the midline without undue force.

Outflare
- Position the hip in flexion and external rotation, increasing outflare
- Have client move the full leg towards the midline against resistance
- Then, on the final move, with the patient fully relaxed, ease the pelvis medially by taking the knee towards the midline without undue force.

Regardless of the corrective procedure, reset symphysis pubis by having the client supine with knees and hips flexed and instruct the client to firmly push the knees together against resistance applied by the massage therapist.

Massage treatment for acute back pain

- Side-lying position is recommended
- If prone, support with pillows under the abdomen and ankles
- *Do not* keep the client in prone position for an extended time – 15 min maximum
- When moving the client from a prone to a side-lying position, have the client slowly assume a hands and knees position, then slowly arch and hunch back (cat/camel move, valley/hill). Then, stretch back towards the heel with arms extended
- Then slowly have him/her move to the side position and bolster for stability
- Target pain control mechanisms
- *Do not* do deep work or any method that causes guarding, flinching or breath holding
- Use rocking, gentle shaking, combined with gliding and kneading to the area of most pain and symptomatic muscle tension
- This will most likely be on the back even though the causal muscle tension and soft tissue problem is usually in the anterior torso
- Massage the hamstring and adductors, gluteals and calves as these are usually short and tight and the firing is out of sequence
- *Do not* attempt to reset firing patterns during acute symptoms
- Turn client supine after working with both left and right sides – bolster under the knees
- The rectus abdominis and pectoralis muscles are likely short and tense
- Use kneading to lengthen these muscles
- Psoas muscles and adductors are likely short and spasming but it is advisable to wait 24–48 h before addressing these muscles
- Continue rocking and shaking.

Subacute treatment using massage

Subacute treatment 24–48 h after onset
- In the context of general massage, repeat acute massage application but begin to address second and third layer muscle shortening, connective tissue pliability and firing patterns
- Use direct inhibition pressure on the psoas, quadratus lumborum, paravertebrals, especially multifidi, always monitoring for guarding response
- *Do not* cause guarding or changes in the breathing
- It is likely that the hip abductors will have tender areas of shortening but lengthen the adductors first
- Gently begin to correct the trunk, gluteal and hamstring firing patterns
- Include massage application for breathing dysfunction since it is commonly associated with low back problems
- Do not over-work or fatigue the client.

Subacute treatment 3–7 days after onset

- Continue with subacute massage application in context of general massage, increasing intensity of the massage as tolerated
- In addition, muscle firing patterns and the short muscles of the upper and lower crossed syndrome need to be normalized
- It is appropriate to gently mobilize the pelvis and ribs
- No pain should be felt during any active or passive movements
- Positional release methods and specific inhibiting pressure can be applied to tender points
- The pressure recreates the symptoms but does not increase the symptoms
- Address trigger points that are most medial, proximal, and painful
- Do not address latent trigger points at this time or work with more than 3–5 areas
- Continue to address breathing function
- The client should be doing gentle stretches and appropriate therapeutic exercises.

Post subacute treatment

- Continue with general massage and address muscles that remain symptomatic
- Begin to assess for body-wide instability, compensation patterns, etc. that are predisposed to an acute back pain event
- Usually, the core muscle firing is weak with synergistic dominance of rectus abdominis and psoas (Chs 4, 5, 6)
- If breathing is dysfunctional, there can be midback pain as well
- Continue to normalize breathing pattern disorder
- For chronic back pain, continue with post subacute treatment and support rehabilitative exercises including breathing retraining (see Ch. 8).

Massage protocol for common back conditions

The protocol offered is only one example of how assessment and treatment of low back dysfunction is integrated into a general massage application. Based on assessment the appropriate methods to treat specific low back pain would be introduced into the massage as is convenient.

FACE AND HEAD

Working with the face is relaxing, therefore, if the face is done first, it can set the stage for a calming massage, or if the face is done at the end of the session, it will gently finish the massage (Fig. 7.22).

- Lightly and systematically stroke the face in multiple directions assessing for temperature, tissue texture changes and tissue ease and bind directions

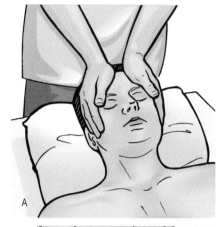
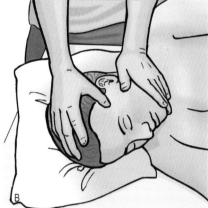
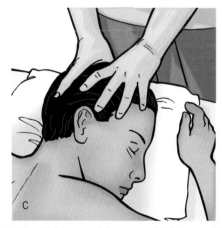

Figure 7.22   (A) Massage of face supine. (B) Massage of face side-lying. (C) Massage of head prone. (From Fritz S 2004 Fundamentals of therapeutic massage, 3rd edn. Mosby, St Louis.)

- To increase circulation to the area of tissue bind and shift neuroresponses, move the skin into multiple directions of ease, and hold the ease position for up to 30–60 s

- Address the muscle structures. Light to moderate compressive force is adequate to address the area
- The muscles that clench the jaw (muscles of mastication) can shorten when a person is stressed
- Stress can cause low back dysfunction and/or the pain experienced from back problems can cause grimacing and stress
- It is prudent to make sure these muscles are functioning normally
- The muscles of mastication often house trigger points
- Hold the tissues housing the trigger point in the ease position using bending forces and move the tissues into bind to stretch the area
- Use gliding and gentle kneading to stretch the areas
- To finish the face, return to the initial light stroking of the lymphatic drain style to support fluid exchange in the area.

General massage of the head begins the assessment process. The connective tissue of the head connects into the lumbo-dorsal fascia. Bind in the connective tissue of the head can also cause bind in the low back. Typically, hair prevents using skin drag palpation methods, however the scalp can be moved into ease and bind positions and the muscles can be palpated for trigger point symptoms. Any soft tissue dysfunctions identified that are appropriate to treat during the massage are most easily addressed with compression methods and then manually stretched using ease and bind movement of the scalp in a connective tissue approach.

- Some clients enjoy having their hair gently stroked and pulled during massage and pulling large bunches of the hair in a slow steady manner can also stretch the tissue
- Compression to the sides of the head and to the front and back coupled with a scratching motion to the scalp can be very pleasant.

NECK

Address this area with the client prone, side-lying and seated (Fig. 7.23).

- Systematically, lightly stroke the area, including assessment methods of scanning and skin drag
- Then, increase the pressure slightly and slowly move the tissue into ease and bind (Fig. 7.24)
- Identify any potential areas that can influence the low back, especially connective tissue structures and tendency to upper and lower crossed syndrome patterns
- Use gliding with a compressive element beginning at the middle of the back of the head at the trapezius attachments and slowly drag the tissue to

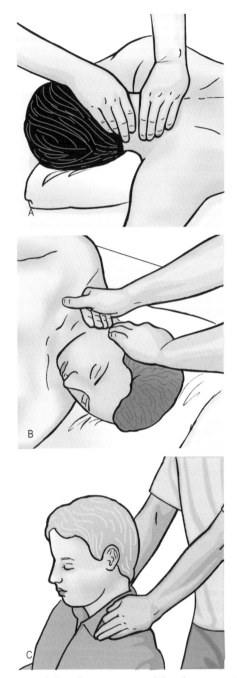

Figure 7.23 (A) Neck massage prone, (B) neck massage side-lying, (C) neck massage seated. (From Fritz S 2004 Fundamentals of therapeutic massage, 3rd edn. Mosby, St Louis.)

the distal attachment of the trapezius at the acromion process and lateral third of the clavicle
- With client prone, begin again at the head and glide towards the acromion

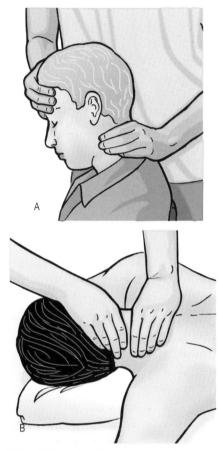

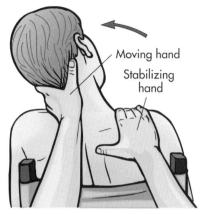

Figure 7.25   Seated position for using muscle energy methods on the neck. (From Fritz S 2004 Fundamentals of therapeutic massage, 3rd edn. Mosby, St Louis.)

Figure 7.24   (A) Seated position for moving tissue of the neck, (B) prone position for moving tissue of the neck. (From Fritz S 2004 Fundamentals of therapeutic massage, 3rd edn. Mosby, St Louis.)

- Then, reverse the direction and work from distal to proximal applying tension force to stretch the area
- Next knead and glide across the muscle fibers, making sure that bending, shear and torsion forces are only sufficient to create a pleasurable sensation while assessing for changes in the tissues
- Use muscle energy methods (Fig. 7.25) and/or direct pressure to inhibit and then stretch short muscles
- Increase intensity of the kneading to further stretch the local tissue if needed and then again apply tension force this time by passively or actively using joint movement and stretching the area
- Integrate specific methods to normalize breathing
- Gentle rocking rhythmic range of motion of the area (oscillation) may be used to continue to relax the area.

TORSO ANTERIOR

When massaging this area, generally target breathing mechanisms. Breathing dysfunction and low back dysfunction are interrelated. The massage therapist influences breathing by maintaining soft tissue mobility in the area and supporting balance between sympathetic and parasympathetic autonomic nervous systems function. This is generally accomplished with a relaxation focus to the general massage.

- This is an appropriate time to assess for trunk flexion firing patterns and then apply corrections as convenient during the massage The pelvis assessments performed supine (as described earlier) can also be incorporated (rotation and flair)
- Massage begins superficially and progresses to deeper tissue layers and then finishes off with superficial work again
- During the massage, various forms of palpation, joint movement and muscle assessment for tissue changes occur
- In general, if soft tissue dysfunctions are identified related to the low back problem as the massage progresses, hold the tissue in ease position until release is felt, or up to 30–60 s, and then the tissues are moved into bind using connective tissue approaches to stretch the tissue
- Use gliding with a compressive element beginning at the shoulder and work from the distal attachment of the pectoralis major (Fig. 7.26) at the arm towards the sternum following fiber direction
- This can be done in supine or side-lying position
- Repeat three or four times each time increasing the drag and moving more slowly

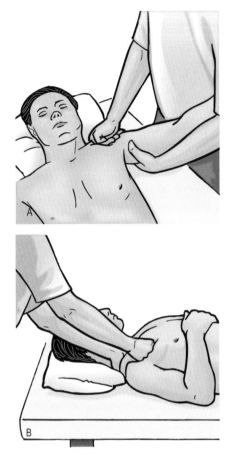

Figure 7.26   Massage of pectoralis major. (From Fritz S 2004 Fundamentals of therapeutic massage, 3rd edn. Mosby, St Louis.)

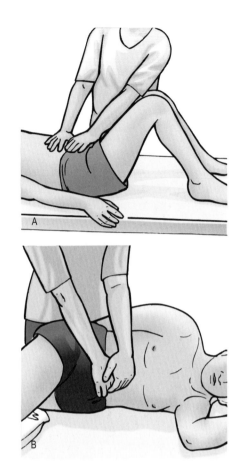

Figure 7.27   (A) Kneading abdominal muscles, supine; (B) kneading abdominal muscles, side-lying. (From Fritz S 2004 Fundamentals of therapeutic massage, 3rd edn. Mosby, St Louis.)

- If short muscles are located, muscle energy methods can be used to facilitate lengthening
- Positional release methods are especially effective for treating various tender points in this area
- Then, reverse the direction and work from distal to proximal applying tension force to stretch the area
- Knead and glide across the muscle fibers, making sure that bending, shear and torsion forces are only sufficient to create a pleasurable sensation while assessing for changes in the tissue
- If the breathing has been dysfunctional for an extended period of time (over 3 months) connective tissue changes are common
- Focused connective tissue massage application is effective

- Once the soft tissue is more normal, then gentle mobilization of the thorax is appropriate
- If the thoracic vertebrae and ribs are restricted, chiropractic or other joint manipulation methods may be appropriate and referral is indicated
- Incorporate all anterior thorax methods for breathing dysfunction
- Move to the abdomen and knead slowly across the fiber direction, as always assessing for dysfunction related to low back issues and then determining appropriateness of treatment based on the history and outcome goals (Fig. 7.27)
- Skin drag palpation is often ticklish in this area so is not used but scanning for heat is possible
- The psoas would be assessed and treated at this time using inhibitory pressure on the muscle belly or by using muscle energy methods and stretching

- Rhythmic compression to the entire anterior torso area stimulates the lymphatic flow, blood circulation and relaxed breathing
- Any areas or functions that received specific treatment should be reassessed for changes.

TORSO POSTERIOR

This area can be addressed in the prone or side-lying position. It is appropriate to assess for hip extension and abduction firing patterns before actually beginning to massage the area and then correction can be incorporated as convenient during the massage. With the client positioned prone, SI joint assessments can be performed and then treatment would be included in the massage as it is convenient.

This area becomes involved in breathing function difficulties as well as low back symptoms.

The muscles commonly problematic are:

- serratus posterior superior and inferior
- levator scapulae
- rhomboids
- latissimus dorsi
- erector spinae and paravertebral especially the multifidi
- quadratus lumborum.

As described previously, massage begins superficially and progresses to deeper layers and then finishes off with superficial work.

- Begin with skin drag palpation and scanning to assess for possible tissue changes related to low back issues
- Use gliding (Fig. 7.28) with a compressive element beginning at the iliac crest and work diagonally along the fibers of the latissimus dorsi ending at the axilla
- Repeat three or four times, each time increasing the drag and moving more slowly to address deeper tissue layers
- Identify areas of tissue bind, heat, increased histamine response and muscle 'knots'
- Move up to the thoracolumbar junction and repeat the same sequence on the lower trapezius (Fig. 7.29)
- Then begin near the tip of the shoulder and glide towards the middle thoracic area to address the middle trapezius
- Repeat three or four times increasing drag (Fig. 7.30) and decreasing speed
- Begin again near the acromion and address the upper trapezius with one or two gliding stokes to complete the surface area

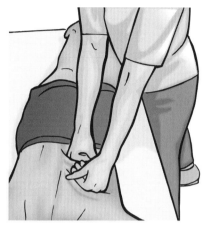

Figure 7.28   Example of gliding with compressive force, prone. (From Fritz S 2004 Fundamentals of therapeutic massage, 3rd edn. Mosby, St Louis.)

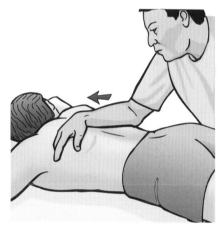

Figure 7.29   Example of gliding with compression using forearm. (From Fritz S 2004 Fundamentals of therapeutic massage, 3rd edn. Mosby, St Louis.)

- Muscle energy methods and stretching (Fig. 7.31) can also be used to address short muscles that relate to the low back condition
- Reverse the direction and work from distal to proximal applying tension force to stretch the area
- Knead (Fig. 7.32) and glide across the muscle fibers, making sure that bending, shear and torsion forces are only sufficient to create a pleasurable sensation while assessing for changes in the tissue
- Increase intensity of the kneading to further stretch the local tissue in the trigger point area and then again apply tension force this time by passively or actively using joint movement and stretching the area

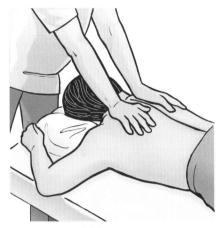

Figure 7.30   Example of gliding with drag on posterior torso. (From Fritz S 2004 Fundamentals of therapeutic massage, 3rd edn. Mosby, St Louis.)

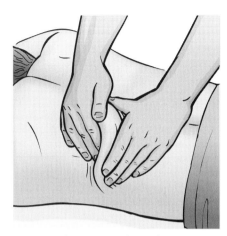

Figure 7.32   Kneading posterior thorax. (From Fritz S 2004 Fundamentals of therapeutic massage, 3rd edn. Mosby, St Louis.)

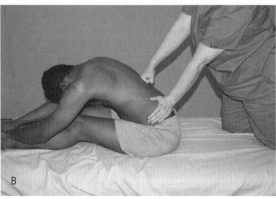

Figure 7.31   (A) Positioning for muscle energy method. (B) Stretching using movement and gliding with drag to affect connective tissue. (Reproduced with kind permission from Mosby's Massage Career Development Series 2006.)

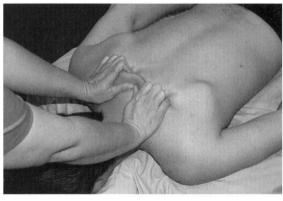

Figure 7.33   Skin rolling along spine. (Reproduced with kind permission from Mosby's Massage Career Development Series 2006.)

- Knead the area again to increase circulation to the area and shift nervous system responses
- Skin roll (Fig 7.33) from the occipital base to the sacrum
- Move the skin into multiple directions of ease, and holding the ease position for up to 30–60 s. If appropriate use lymphatic drain methods in the area
- Gentle rhythmic rocking within the ranges of motion of the area (oscillation) may be used to continue to relax the area
- Identify rigidity in the ribs with the client prone bilaterally (on both sides of the spine) at the facet joints beginning near the seventh cervical vertebra and moving down towards the lower ribs maintaining compressive force near the facet joints

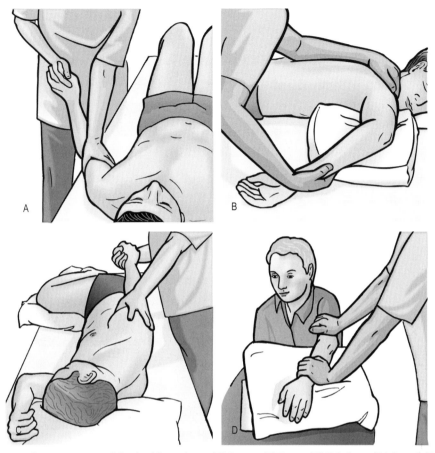

Figure 7.34   Positions for moving tissue of the shoulder and arm. (A) Supine. (B) Prone. (C) Side-lying. (D) Seated. (From Fritz S 2004 Fundamentals of therapeutic massage, 3rd edn. Mosby, St Louis.)

- If an area identified relates to the low back issue, treat with various muscle energy techniques
- Rhythmic compression to the area stimulates various aspects of fluid movement, supports relaxed breathing and finishes the massage of the area
- Any areas or function that received specific intervention should be reassessed for changes.

SHOULDER, ARM AND HAND

The area is massaged in supine, prone side-lying and seated positions. Massage of the torso and neck naturally progresses to the shoulder, arm and hand. All assessment methods described in Chapter 4 can be incorporated during the massage application. The most common muscle in this area related to low back problems is the latissimus dorsi. It is often short and various methods can be used to inhibit the muscle and then stretch it. During the general massage, tissue is assessed for low back issues relating to any symptoms the client may have.

- Commencing with the client prone, massage begins superficially, progresses to deeper layers and then finishes off with superficial work
- Finish the area with kneading, compression and gliding
- To increase circulation to the area and shift nervous system responses, move the skin into multiple directions of ease, and hold the ease position for up to 30–60 s
- Then move the tissue into bind to stretch the area
- Stretch the area with either active or passive joint movement or direct tissue application incorporating gliding and kneading, whichever is more effective. It is also appropriate to use a combination of stretching methods (Fig. 7.34).

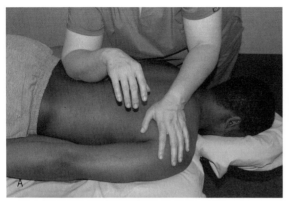
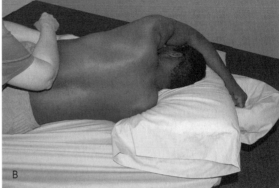

Figure 7.35 Massage of lumbar area, (A) prone, (B) side-lying. (Reproduced with kind permission from Mosby's Massage Career Development Series 2006.)

The intrinsic muscles of the hand are addressed next.

- Systematically work the area, using compression and gliding of the soft tissue between the fingers, the web of the thumb and on the palm that opposes the thumb and little finger
- There is also a network of lymphatic vessels in the palm that when rhythmically compressed assists lymphatic movement.

LOW BACK AND HIP

This area would be a major target area of the massage for managing low back pain and dysfunction. The low back and hip area is massaged in prone and side-lying positions (Fig. 7.35).

Massage of the torso naturally progresses to the low back and hip area. If there are indications of pelvic distortion patterns, it may be prudent to use massage to normalize hamstrings, quadratus lumborum, tensor fascia latae and piriformis.

- Massage begins superficially and progresses to deeper layers and then finishes off with superficial work
- Systematically, lightly stroke the area. This is the assessment of tissue changes related to low back issues
- Various firing pattern assessments, strength testing for muscle weakness and SI joint assessments can be performed at this time, if not previously done
- To increase circulation to the area and shift nervous system responses, move the skin into multiple directions of ease, and hold the ease position for up to 30–60 s
- Methods of lymphatic drainage are also appropriate if edema is present

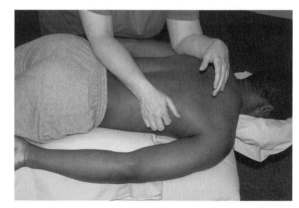

Figure 7.36 Compressive gliding from shoulder to opposite hip. (Reproduced with kind permission from Mosby's Massage Career Development Series 2006.)

- Increase the pressure slightly
- Begin on the posterior to address the lumbar region that connects with the hip
- This area was addressed while massaging the torso but now is massaged in relationship to the low back and hip
- Carry the strokes into the gluteus maximus
- Repeat with the latissimus dorsi again in relation to low back function. Begin at the shoulder and carry the stroke all the way into the opposite gluteus maximus (Fig. 7.36)
- Systematically repeat the gliding, interspersing with kneading to assess the deeper tissue layers for trigger point symptoms, or the tell-tale knots that refer pain in trigger point patterns, SI joint dysfunction, quadratus dysfunction and any other low back concerns. Palpate for sacral tender points

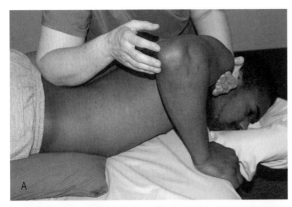

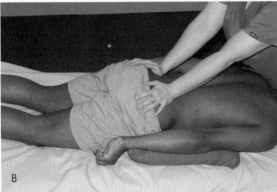

Figure 7.37 (A) Example of compression with shear force. (B) Example of stretching after compression. (Reproduced with kind permission from Mosby's Massage Career Development Series 2006.)

- If trigger or tender points are identified, address with the least invasive method of skin ease and bind movement or skin rolling
- Progress to compression methods with positional release. As a last resort, if there are connective tissue changes, shear forces introduced with friction can be used (Fig. 7.37)
- Stretch the area with direct tissue methods by kneading and slow gliding and connective tissue methods. MET and stretching are also options
- Lymphatic drainage methods support fluid movement in the area
- Finish by gliding and kneading the entire area.

THE THIGHS, LEGS AND FEET

The area can be massaged in all basic positions (Fig. 7.38). Massage of the area naturally progresses from the hip. As with other body regions, massage begins superficially, progresses to deeper layers and then finishes off with superficial work.

- To increase circulation to the area and shift nervous system responses, move the skin into multiple directions of ease, and hold the ease position for up to 30–60 s
- Increase the pressure slightly again gliding and kneading the entire area. Systematically repeat the gliding interspersing with kneading to assess the deeper tissue for tissue changes and treat appropriately
- If there are connective tissue changes, shear forces introduced with friction can be used. Stretch the area with direct tissue methods by kneading and slow gliding and connective tissue methods
- The hamstrings, quadriceps and adductor muscles are all factors if low back pain is present
- Assess to determine if these muscles are short, weak, or activating inappropriately (usually hamstring and erector spinae are overactive due to inhibited gluteus maximus)
- Move the hip and knee passively through flexion, extension, internal and external rotation to assess for restrictions in joint function
- Trigger point activity can be addressed with compression and muscle energy methods. Binding at the joint can be addressed with indirect functional methods (move into ease and hold for up to 60 s and then move into bind and the stretch just beyond bind) and connective tissue methods
- Use active and passive joint movement (Fig. 7.39) to reassess the area
- Lymphatic drainage methods support fluid movement in the area
- Finish by gliding and kneading the entire area
- Add gentle shaking and oscillation in various positions.

The intrinsic muscles of the foot are addressed next.

- Side-lying is the best position
- Work systematically using compression and gliding of the soft tissue of the sole of the foot (Fig. 7.40)
- There is also a network of lymphatic vessels in the sole of the feet that, when rhythmically compressed, will assist lymphatic movement
- To finish off, use gentle shaking and oscillation and compression and passive movement.

RE-EVALUATION

The specific areas addressed during massage should be re-evaluated for results and this information incorporated into the plan for the next massage session. Use the same methods for revaluation as were used for initial assessment.

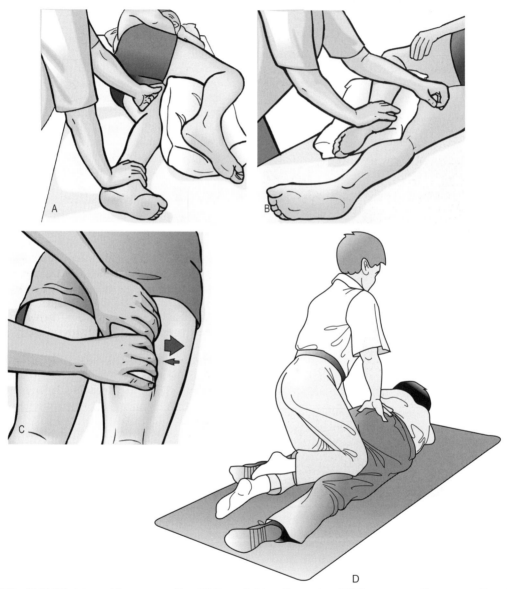

Figure 7.38 (A,B) Side-lying position massage of leg. (C) Prone shaking of hamstrings. (D) Compression of hamstrings. (From Fritz S 2004 Fundamentals of therapeutic massage, 3rd edn. Mosby, St Louis.)

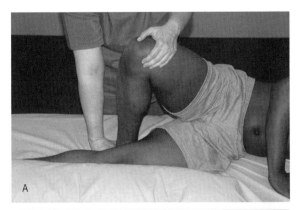

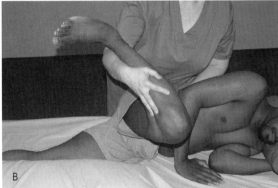

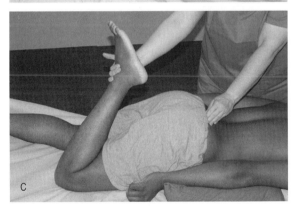

Figure 7.39   Examples of joint movement of the hip and knee. (Reproduced with kind permission from Mosby's Massage Career Development Series 2006.)

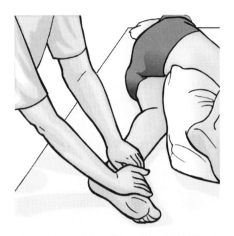

Figure 7.40   Massage of foot. (From Fritz S 2004 Fundamentals of therapeutic massage, 3rd edn. Mosby, St Louis.)

Massage and prevention of low back pain:

- Massage may be one of the most effective measures for preventing low back dysfunction
- Massage can address causal factors before they become serious enough to cause back pain

- General full body massage that incorporates application to the various tissue types and layers of soft tissue may shift the circulation and metabolic dysfunction to a more normal state
- Muscles with the tendency to form soft tissue dysfunctions can be maintained in a more pliable and lengthened state
- The soft tissue is regularly searched for changes during general massage and the soft tissue can be normalized before the trigger point develops, becomes fibrotic, or sets up satellite points
- Tendency to postural distortion from non-optimal use patterns during work or daily and recreational activities can be managed. Massage can also help maintain a more normal breathing pattern and autonomic nervous system balance
- For massage to be effective, the person would need to have massage on a regular basis, with weekly sessions ideal and at the minimum a monthly massage
- The basic prevention strategy for back problems is to develop a strong back. Since most injuries are due to muscle weakness, increased strength is the answer to almost every back problem.
- Strengthening the core is essential
- Stamina is equally important, strength is not enough, and the Chapter 8 will discuss this in more depth.

KEY POINTS

- Massage can be an effective approach to incorporating and blending various assessment and treatment options for low back pain
- Massage is generally enjoyed by clients/patients so compliance with treatment may be increased
- Massage can be a satisfactory treatment option for symptom management if the client/patient will not make the behavior changes necessary to address causal factors
- Massage for low back pain is an outcome based process that incorporates many different modalities and methods to achieve the goals identified including pain management, increased mobility and normalization of soft tissue structure and function
- To implement an outcome based massage application, it is necessary to perform appropriate assessments to target massage

- Massage can be generically explained by describing qualities of touch and application of mechanical forces to influence the body's structure and function
- Generalized full body massage application can ease low back symptoms. These include pain management, connective tissue normalization and breathing function normalization
- Specific massage strategies can address local dysfunctional areas such as short muscles, altered firing patterns and areas of fibrosis and adhesion and joint dysfunction
- Massage methods for acute back pain are more general and less specific than methods for chronic back pain
- Massage focused for chronic back pain is both symptom management and reversal of causal factors
- Massage is an effective aspect of a program to prevent low back pain.

References

Chaitow L, Bradley D, Gilbert C 2002 Multidisciplinary approaches to breathing pattern disorders. Churchill Livingstone, Edinburgh

De Domenico G, Wood E 1997 Beard's massage, 4th edn. WB Saunders, Philadelphia

Freeman L W, Lawlis G F 2001 Mosby's complementary and alternative medicine, a research-based approach. Mosby, St Louis

Fritz S 2004 Fundamentals of therapeutic massage, 3rd edn. Mosby/Elsevier, St Louis

Gehlsen G, Ganion L, Helfst R 1999 Fibroblast responses to variation in soft tissue mobilization pressure. Medicine and Science in Sports and Exercise 31(4):531–535

Lederman E 1997 Fundamentals of manual therapy physiology, neurology, and psychology. Churchill Livingstone, New York

Mosby's Massage Career Development Series 2006

NCCAM 2004 Manipulative and body-based practices: An overview. Publication No. D238, October. Online. Available: http://www.nccam.nih.gov; e-mail: info@nccam.nih.gov Aug 2005

Wieting J M, Cugalj A P, Kaplan R J, Talavera F 2005 Massage, traction, and manipulation. Online. Available: http//www.eMedicine.com Aug 2005

Yahia L H, Pigeon P, DesRosiers E A 1993 Viscoelastic properties of the human lumbodorsal fascia. Journal of Biomedical Engineering 15(5):425–429

Yates J 2004 A physician's guide to therapeutic massage, 3rd edn. Curties-Overzet, Toronto

Chapter 8

Prevention and rehabilitation: core stability and breathing retraining

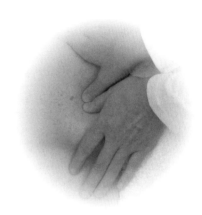

The requirements for preventing low back injury have been summarized by Liebenson (2000a) as:

- 'Conditioning or adaptation', i.e. avoiding undue stress and improvement of flexibility and stability, leading to greater tolerance to strain
- He also suggests that there is evidence that too little (or infrequent) tissue stress can be damaging, as can too much (or too frequent, or prolonged) exposure to biomechanical stress. In other words, deconditioning through inactivity provokes dysfunction just as efficiently as does excessive and inappropriate biomechanical stress
- McGill (1998) suggests that a neutral spine should be used in all loading tasks to reduce the chance of injury. He also warns that it is important to avoid bending and stooping to lift
- Additional common sense methods are suggested, including rotation of tasks to vary loads, introduction of frequent short rest breaks, and maintaining loads close to the spine when lifting (McGill & Norman 1993)
- Particular caution is needed at vulnerable times (for the spine), after long periods of rest, for example early morning soon after rising from bed, and after sitting for 30 min or more (Adams et al 1987).

CORE STABILIZATION ASSESSMENT AND EXERCISES

Both the abdominal musculature and the trunk extensors are important in restoring stability to the spine (Cholewicki & McGill 1996, Liebenson 2000b).

A variety of exercises have been developed to achieve core stability involving the corset of muscles which surround, stabilize and, to an extent, move the lumbar spine, such as transversus abdominis, the abdominal oblique muscles, diaphragm, erector spinae, multifidi, etc.

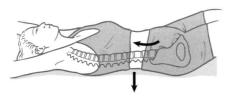

Figure 8.1 'Neutral spine' coordination test. (Reproduced with permission from Journal of Bodywork and Movement Therapies 2000; 4(2):110.)

Basic 'dead-bug' exercise/test

A 'coordination' test that assists in evaluating the patient's ability to maintain the lumbar spine in a steady state during different degrees of loading has been developed. This 'dead-bug' exercise (Richardson et al 1999) easily becomes a core stability exercise if repeated regularly.

- The patient adopts a supine hook-lying position, with a pressure (bio)feedback pad (inflatable cushion attached to pressure gauge, similar to the unit used to test blood pressure) under the lumbar spine
- The inflated pad registers the degree of pressure being applied by the lumbar spine towards the floor. The objective is to maintain the pressure throughout the performance of various degrees of activity, all the while maintaining normal breathing (Figs 8.1, 8.2A–G)
- First, the patient is asked to hollow the back, bringing the umbilicus towards the spine/floor, so initiating co-contraction of transversus abdominis and multifidus, and to maintain this position as increasing degrees of load are applied by either:
  1. Gradually straightening one leg by sliding the heel along the floor: This causes the hip flexors to work eccentrically and, if this over-rides the stability of the pelvis, it will tilt. Therefore, if there is a change (reduction) in pressure on the gauge or if a pelvic tilting/increased lumbar lordosis is observed or palpated before the leg is fully extended, this suggests *deep abdominal muscular insufficiency* involving transversus abdominis and internal obliques.
  2. Once the basic stabilization exercise of hollowing the abdomen – while maintaining pressure to the floor – is achievable *without the breath being held*, more advanced stabilization exercises may be introduced.
  3. These involve, in a graduated way, introducing variations on lower limb or trunk loading, and

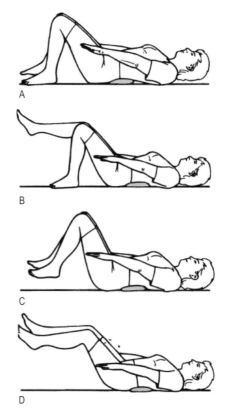

Figure 8.2 (A–D) Neutral spine coordination test with added load. (Reproduced with permission from Journal of Bodywork and Movement Therapies 2000; 4(2):111.)

are performed while maintaining the lumbar spine pressed towards the floor (confirmed by a relatively constant reading on the pressure gauge or by observation). See examples of exercises later in this chapter for an evolution of increasing difficulty.

4. These graduated stabilization exercises involve the adoption by the patient of positions which progress as illustrated in Figure 8.2A–G.
5. As well as abdominal tone and stability, it is necessary to encourage extensor function to be optimal and coordinated with abdominal muscle function. The 'superman' pose (below) encourages this.

Warm-up first

To encourage spinal extensor tone and strength, in order to encourage spinal and 'core' stability, simple home exercise protocols are suggested.

The exercises described below, for encouraging stability, are safe. Ideally, these should be performed after warming-up and not immediately in the morning or after prolonged sitting (Green et al 2002).

Note: Ideally, whoever teaches these to patients should be trained in exercise physiology, or be a Pilates trainer, or equivalent.

Abdominal bracing

This involves co-activation of muscles 360° around the lumbar spine during performance of all/any of these exercises. It involves a light contraction, using no more than 10% of available strength (the amount of contractile effort that you would use if you were being tickled) (McGill 2002, McGill et al 2003).

It is absolutely essential to the effectiveness of this that the person performing the exercise does not hold the breath while bracing the trunk muscles.

The *cat-camel exercise* is an ideal way to warm-up the spine. It is not a stretch but teaches the spine and associated muscles to move in a coordinated way.

Instructions to patient:

- Kneel on a carpeted floor so that the weight is taken on your flexed knees and elbows
- Your thighs should be at right-angles to the floor
- To focus on mobilizing the upper thoracic spine, have the elbows level with your ears
- Breathe in deeply and arch your back upward as far as is possible, allowing your head to drop towards the floor, rounding the thoracic spine.
- Try to imagine that, as this is being done, your navel is being pulled upwards to meet the spine, thus effectively increasing the degree of arching (and increasing stability) (Fig. 8.3A)
- After holding your breath for 5 s, release it and simultaneously start to lower your thoracic spine towards the floor, while also raising the head (Fig. 8.3B)
- This effectively flattens and depresses your thoracic spine
- Hold this position for 5 s before inhaling and arching again

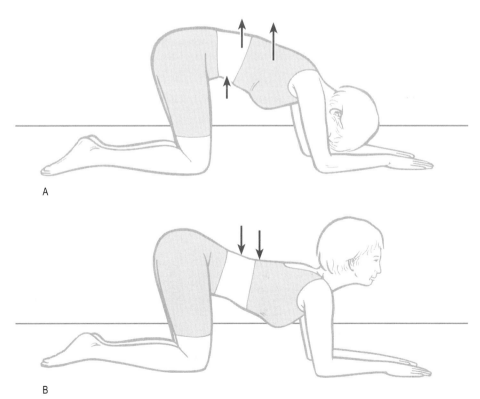

A

B

Figure 8.3   Positions for spinal mobilization. (A) Camel (B) Cat. (From Chaitow 2003.)

- Repeat the 'cat/camel' exercise five or six times in each direction
- In order to localize the effect of this mobilization at the junction of the lumbar and thoracic spine, your hands – rather than the elbows – should be used for floor support
- All other aspects of the procedure remain the same.

Performing this mobilizing sequence is ideal before doing core stability exercises.

The **'superman' pose**, also known as the 'quadruped leg reach', teaches control of a 'neutral' spine during periods of limb motion (Fig. 8.4).

Instructions to patient:

- Kneel on all fours, balanced on your hands and lower legs, spine straight
- Introduce the braced abdomen contraction
- Extend one leg behind you (you are now balanced on two hands and one lower leg), gradually raising it until it is level with your waist
- Hold this for 5 s
- Maintain your 'braced abdomen' and a straight spine throughout, and breathe normally and slowly
- Lower the leg and repeat until you start to find it difficult
- Now do precisely same with the other leg raised until you start to feel difficulty
- When you can perform each of these 12 times, add the next progression, which involves raising one leg as above, as well as *the opposite* arm (a sort of 'superman' position)
- Once you can raise the right arm and left leg, as well as the left arm and right leg, 12 times, for 5 s each, while maintaining a 'braced abdomen', you will be sure to have toned your multifidi to an excellent state of endurance.

The key to performing this is avoiding any twist of the spine, or lumbar hyperextension.

More advanced stability exercises

Motor control or stability training requires an emphasis on endurance rather than strength (Richardson et al

1999). These exercises should be repeated (Brügger 1960), eight, then six times. Each exercise should be performed slowly with a prolonged isometric hold time.

They should be performed twice a day for up to 3 months to achieve optimal results. Learning to coordinate breathing while simultaneously bracing is one of the key skills to be learned. The *side bridge* is an excellent, safe way to train the lateral oblique musculature (for side bridge on knees, see Fig. 8.5).

Instructions to patient:

- Lie on your side with legs flexed at the knee, one on the other
- Use the forearm that is resting on the floor to raise you sideways until your hips are off the floor, and your body is in a straight line (i.e. no sagging)
- Your free arm should either lie alongside your trunk, or be crossed over the chest so that the hand can rest on the opposite shoulder
- Keep breathing normally all the time
- Normal holding time for young healthy individuals (early 20s) should be 60 s for males, and 40 s for females
- Alternatively, see whether you can perform 10 repetitions of raising yourself into this position, and holding for 5 s before lowering and repeating.

The abdominals can be trained with the *supported dead bug*, where one foot stays on the floor as the other is moved/raised, progressing (when this is easy to

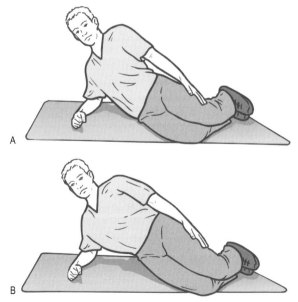

A

B

Figure 8.5   Side bridge on knees. (A) Start position. (B) Final position. (After Liebenson 2004.)

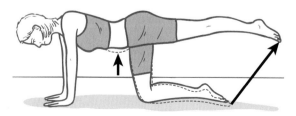

Figure 8.4   Quadruped leg reach. (After Liebenson 2004.)

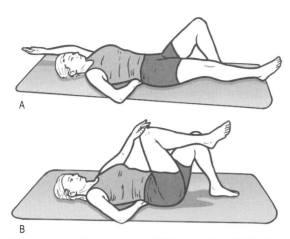

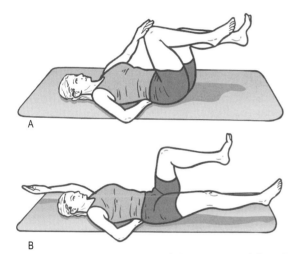

Figure 8.6   Dead bug supported. (A) Start position. (B) Final position (After Liebenson 2004.)

Figure 8.7   Dead bug unsupported. (A) Start position. (B) Final position. (After Liebenson 2004.)

perform) to *unsupported dead-bug* where neither foot is on the floor (Figs 8.6, 8.7).

A further progression involves a *partial curl-up* with spinal neutral control (slight lordosis).

Instructions to patient:

- Lie on your back, hips bent to 45°, knees bent to 90°, feet flat on the floor (or with one knee flexed and the other leg straight) and with hands behind your back, elbows touching the floor (Fig. 8.8)
- Brace your core muscles by bearing down slightly, without holding your breath
- Slowly raise your head and shoulders from the floor, and then slowly round your back as you curl up further

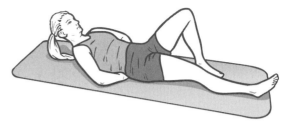

Figure 8.8   Trunk curl-up. (After Liebenson 2004.)

- Stay in this position as you breathe in and out slowly, twice
- Be careful not to poke your chin forwards, and keep your elbows on the floor
- If you feel any strain in the back when doing this, stop, lie down again, brace the abdomen against the spine and start again
- Slowly roll down again, without arching your back and repeat for a total of 12 times
- When this is easy to perform, do the same exercise but when you have introduced the curl, lift your elbows from the floor.

Brügger's relief position

Brügger's relief position for postural and breathing rehabilitation (Brügger 1960, Lewit 1999) reverses many of the stresses caused during long periods of sitting, facilitating muscles which tend to inhibition, and inhibiting muscles which tend to shortening (Fig. 8.9).

These are the instructions that should be given to the patient:

1   Sit close to the edge of a chair ('perch'), with your arms hanging down, palms facing forward
2   Place your feet directly below knees, which are apart and lower than the hips
3   Your feet should be turned slightly outward, with ankles directly below the knees
4   As you slowly exhale, let your pelvis roll back and allow the spine to fall into 'C'-shape
5   The neck and head should follow the spinal curve
6   As you inhale, roll your pelvis slightly forward to produce a *small* degree of arching of the lower back
7   As the spine slightly extends, easing the sternum slightly forward and up, allow your neck, head and eyes to follow the spinal curve, chin in
8   At same time, turn your arms outward, until the thumbs face slightly backwards
9   Exhale as you repeat the process, slightly rounding your back, and inhale as you slightly arch your back and turn the arms outward.

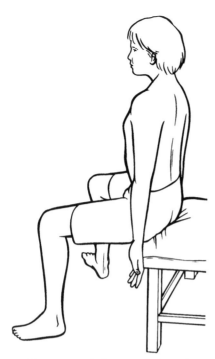

Figure 8.9   The Brügger relief position. (After Liebenson, from Chaitow 2003.)

Repeat the entire process several times a day at least and whenever you sense muscle tension, or feel a need for deeper breathing.

BREATHING REHABILITATION

It has been established that disturbed breathing patterns have a negative effect on core stability, motor control, balance and pain perception (Balaban & Thayer 2001, Hodges & Richardson 1999). Learning better breathing can enhance better spinal function (the diaphragm is a major part of the spinal support system) (Loeppky et al 2001).

Breathing pattern disorders affect large numbers of people, mainly female (Hodges et al 2001) – partly because of progesterone, a respiratory accelerator it is thought – and evidence suggests that a combination of retraining exercises, education and appropriate bodywork (see suggestions below) can help normalize the majority of such problems, over a period of months (Aust & Fischer 1997, Han et al 1996).

Retraining essentials

Breathing retraining requires a combination of elements that also seem to operate in postural retraining (such as the Alexander technique):

- *Understanding* the processes: a cognitive, intellectual, awareness of the mechanisms and issues involved in breathing pattern disorders
- Retraining exercises that include aspects that operate *subcortically*, allowing replacement of currently habituated patterns with more appropriate ones
- Biomechanical *structural modifications* that remove obstacles to desirable and necessary functional changes
- *Time* for these elements to merge and become incorporated into moment-to-moment use patterns.

Pursed lip breathing

Pursed lip breathing (Faling 1995, Tisp et al 1986), combined with diaphragmatic breathing, enhances pulmonary efficiency.

- The patient is seated or supine with the dominant hand on the abdomen and the other hand on the chest
- The patient is asked to breathe in through the nose and out through the mouth, with pursed lips, ensuring diaphragmatic involvement by means of movement of the abdomen against the hand on inhalation
- Exhalation through the pursed lips is performed slowly, and has been shown to relieve dyspnea, slow the respiratory rate, increase tidal volume, and to help restore diaphragmatic function
- Thirty or more cycles should be repeated morning and evening as part of the anti-arousal exercise, see below.

Anti-arousal breathing

Patient's instructions for anti-arousal breathing (Cappo & Holmes 1984, Grossman et al 1985) are as follows:

1 Sit or recline comfortably, and exhale slowly and fully *through pursed lips*
2 Imagine a candle flame about 6 in from your mouth and blow a thin stream of air at it
3 As you exhale, count silently to establish the length of the outbreath
4 When you have exhaled fully, without strain, pause for a count of 'one', then inhale through the nose. Full exhalation creates a 'coiled spring', making inhalation easier
5 Count to yourself to establish how long your in-breath lasts
6 Without pausing to hold the breath, exhale slowly and fully, through pursed lips, blowing the air in a thin stream, and pause for a count of one
7 Repeat the inhalation and exhalation for not less than 30 cycles (morning and evening)

8   After some weeks of daily practice, you should achieve an inhalation phase which lasts 2–3 s, and an exhalation phase of 6–7 s, without strain

9   Exhalation should always be slow and continuous, there is little value in breathing the air out in 2 s and then simply waiting until the count reaches eight before inhaling again

10 Practice twice daily, and repeat the exercise for a few minutes (6 cycles takes about 1 min) every hour if you feel anxious, or when stress or pain increases

11 Practice on waking, and before bedtime, and if at all possible before meals

12 Always incorporate methods that reduce over-activity of neck/shoulder muscles, as described below.

Inhibiting shoulder rise during breathing retraining

When applying breathing retraining it is important to teach tactics that restrict over-activity of the accessory breathing muscles, in order to reduce 'shoulder rising' on inhalation. The methods might include:

- Pushing elbows/forearms onto arms of the chair, on inhalation (Fig. 8.10A)

- Arms behind back, grasping wrist with other hand and pulling down, on inhalation (Fig. 8.10B)
- Reclining with hands behind head ('beach pose') to open chest and reduce shoulder movement (Fig. 8.10C)
- Interlocking hands on lap and applying finger-pad pressure to dorsum of hands, on inhalation, to inhibit shoulder movement
- Adopting Brügger's relief position throughout breathing exercises (see above).

Suggested manual treatment sequence for breathing pattern disorder (BPD) problems

Treatment and retraining commonly involves 12 weekly sessions, followed by treatment sessions every 2–3 weeks, to approximately 6 months.

An educational component should be included at each session.

First two sessions (not less than weekly)
- Upper fixators/accessory breathing muscles (upper trapezii, levator, scalenes/SCS, pectorals, latissimus dorsi) release/stretch, plus attention to trigger points

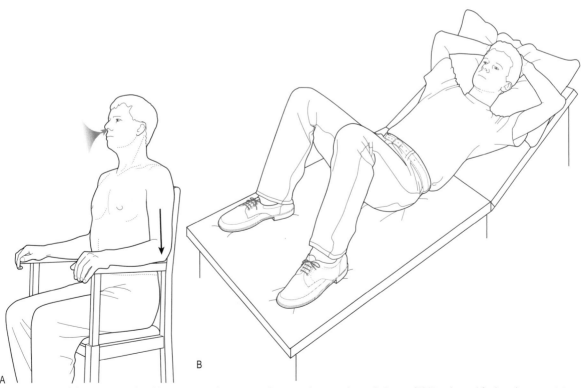

Figure 8.10   (A) Restricting shoulder movement by pressing forearms downward on inhalation. (B) 'Beach pose' for breathing retraining (after Bradley).

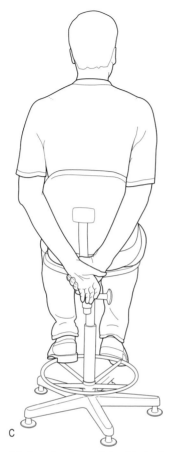

C

Figure 8.10 (C) Seated with arms behind back allows restriction of shoulder movement on inhalation (after Bradley). (From Chaitow 2003.)

- Diaphragm area (anterior intercostals, sternum, abdominal attachments costal margin, quadratus lumborum, psoas) release/stretch, plus attention to trigger points
- *Retraining*: pursed lip breathing/control pause/restricting tendency for shoulder rise with upper chest pattern.

Sessions 3 and 4 (weeks)
- As above, plus mobilization of thoracic spine and rib articulations (plus lymphatic pump)
- Address fascial and osseous links (cranial, pelvic, lower extremity)
- *Retraining*: anti-arousal breathing pattern, plus specific relaxation methods (autogenics, visualization, meditation, etc.), stress management.

Sessions 5–12 (weeks)
- As above, plus other body influences (ergonomics, posture)
- *Retraining*: additional exercises as appropriate.

Weeks 13–26
- Review and treat residual dysfunctional patterns/tissues
- Plus, as indicated: nutrition, counseling, stress management.

Adjunctive methods used throughout as applicable: hydrotherapy, tai chi, yoga, Pilates, massage, acupuncture.

KEY POINTS

- Core stability is a central element of prevention and rehabilitation
- All core stability exercises ('dead-bug', 'superman', 'side-bridge', etc.) should be performed with abdominal and low back muscles 'braced', using no more than 10% of muscle strength
- During performance of all core stability exercises with braced trunk muscles, it is essential that the individual maintains normal breathing, and not a held breath
- A warm-up is helpful before performance of core stability exercises (e.g. 'cat-camel')
- Brügger's relief position offers an excellent way of easing stressed postural muscles and encouraging better breathing
- Breathing rehabilitation is a key aspect of back rehabilitation
- Postural and/or breathing rehabilitation take time: 3–6 months, as old habits are altered
- Breathing rehabilitation involves a combination of breathing exercises (e.g. 'pursed-lip' breathing) as well as reduction of excessive accessory muscle activity, plus bodywork to mobilize the structures of the breathing mechanism
- The bodywork element of breathing retraining focuses on mobilization of the thorax (ribs, etc.) as well as releasing and stretching (where appropriate) shortened muscles associated with breathing, such as upper fixators of the shoulder, diaphragm, psoas and quadratus lumborum
- Trigger point deactivation may also be required.

References

Adams M, Dolan P, Hutton W 1987 Diurnal variations in the stresses on the lumbar spine. Spine 12(2):130–137

Aust G, Fischer K 1997 Changes in body equilibrium response caused by breathing. A posturographic study with visual feedback. Laryngorhinootologie 76(10):577–582

Balaban C, Thayer J 2001 Neurological bases for balance-anxiety links. Journal of Anxiety Disorders 15(1–2):53–79

Brügger A 1960 Pseudoradikulare syndrome. Acta Rheumatologica 18:1

Cappo B, Holmes D 1984 Utility of prolonged respiratory exhalation for reducing physiological and psychological arousal in non-threatening and threatening situations. Journal of Psychosomatic Research 28(4):265–273

Chaitow L 2003 Maintaining body balance, flexibility and stability. Churchill Livingstone, Edinburgh

Chaitow L, DeLany J 2002 Clinical applications of neuromuscular technique, Volume 2. Churchill Livingstone, Edinburgh

Cholewicki J, McGill S 1996 Mechanical stability of the in vivo lumbar spine. Clinical Biomechanics 11:1–15

Faling L 1995 Controlled breathing techniques and chest physical therapy in chronic obstructive pulmonary disease. In: Casabur R (ed.) Principles and practices of pulmonary therapy. WB Saunders, Philadelphia

Green J, Grenier S, McGill S M 2002 Low back stiffness is altered with warmup and bench rest: Implications for athletes. Medicine and Science in Sports and Exercise 34(7):1076–1081

Grossman P, de Swart J C, Defares P B 1985 A controlled study of breathing therapy for treatment of hyperventilation syndrome. Journal of Psychosomatic Research 29(1):49–58

Han J, Stegen K, De Valck C et al 1996 Influence of breathing therapy on complaints, anxiety and breathing pattern in patients with hyperventilation syndrome and anxiety disorders. Journal of Psychosomatic Research 41(5):481–493

Hodges P, Heinjnen I, Gandevia S 2001 Postural activity of the diaphragm is reduced in humans when respiratory demand increases. Journal of Physiology 537(3):999–1008

Hodges P, Richardson C 1999 Altered trunk muscle recruitment in people with low back pain with upper limb movement at different speeds. Archives of Physical Medicine Rehabilitation 80:1005–1012

Lewit K 1999 Manipulative therapy in rehabilitation of the locomotor system, 3rd edn. Butterworths, London

Liebenson C 2000a The quadratus lumborum and spinal stability. Journal of Bodywork and Movement Therapies 4(1):49–54

Liebenson C 2000b The trunk extensors and spinal stability. Journal of Bodywork and Movement Therapies 4(4):246–249

Liebenson C 2000c Advice for the clinician: the role of the transverse abdominis in promoting spinal stability. Journal of Bodywork and Movement Therapies 4(2):109–112

Liebenson C 2004 Spinal stabilization – an update. Part 3 – training. Journal of Bodywork and Movement Therapies 8(4):278–285

Loeppky J, Scotto P, Charlton G et al 2001 Ventilation is greater in women than men, but the increase during acute altitude hypoxia is the same. Respiration Physiology 125(3):225–237

McGill S M 1998 Low back exercises: prescription for the healthy back. In: ACSM (ed.) Resources manual for guidelines for exercise testing and prescription, 3rd edn. American College of Sports Medicine, Williams and Wilkins, Baltimore

McGill S M 2002 Low back disorders: Evidence based prevention and rehabilitation. Human Kinetics Publishers, Champaign

McGill S, Grenier S, Bluhm M 2003 Previous history of LBP with work loss is related to lingering deficits in biomechanical, physiological, personal, psychosocial and motor control characteristics. Ergonomics 46:731–746

McGill S, Norman R 1993 Low back biomechanics in industry. In: Grabiner M (ed.) Current issues in biomechanics. Human Kinetics, Champaign

Richardson C, Jull G, Hides J, Hodges P 1999 Therapeutic exercise for spinal segmental stabilisation in low back pain. Churchill Livingstone, Edinburgh

Tisp B, Burns M, Kro D et al 1986 Pursed lip breathing using ear oximetry. Chest 90:218–222

Chapter 9

Prevention

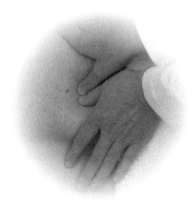

If prevention is to be meaningful, then the basic causes of back pain should be avoided. This is, however, not always possible as congenital, in-born, features may be key features of the background to back problems. Additionally, a history of overuse, misuse and abuse (trauma) often accompanied by disuse may be beyond current influence. It is within that context that the present situation needs to be viewed, with as many factors that are capable of removal, improvement, reduction being attended to while at the same time functional improvement is initiated through exercise and therapeutic endeavor (Janda 1984). While there are many treatment methods that have been shown to reduce pain, for prevention of chronic pain, exercise is the proven best choice. Therefore, as soon as possible, self-treatment with exercise should be recommended.

HOW VULNERABLE IS THE PATIENT?

Single leg stance balance test

This is a reliable procedure (Bohannon et al 1984) for information regarding vulnerability/stability as well as for retraining. Fortunately, it requires no equipment other than a timer (Fig. 9.1).

Procedure
- The patient is instructed to raise one foot up without touching it to the support leg
- The knee can be raised to any comfortable height
- The patient is asked to balance for up to 30 s with eyes open
- After testing standing on one leg, the other should be tested
- When single leg standing with eyes open is successful for 30 s, the patient is asked to 'spot' something on a wall opposite, and to then close the eyes while visualizing that spot
- An attempt is made to balance for 30 s.

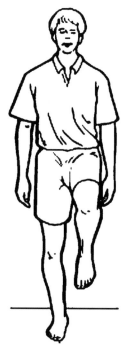

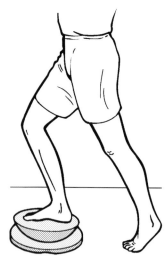

Figure 9.2   Wobble board as used in balance retraining (available from OPTP (800) 367 7393 USA). (From Chaitow 2003.)

 Figure 9.1   Single-leg stance balance test. (Reproduced from Liebenson CS. Advice for clinician and patient: sensory-motor training. Journal for Bodywork and Movement Therapies 5(1):21–28, 2001).

Scoring

The time is recorded when any of the following occurs:

- The raised foot touches the ground or more than lightly touches the other leg
- The stance foot changes (shifts) position or toes rise
- There is hopping on the stance leg
- The hands touch anything other than the person's own body.

By regularly (daily) practicing this balance exercise, the time achieved in balance with eyes closed will increase. Over time, more challenging balance exercises can be introduced, including the use of wobble boards and balance sandals (Figs 9.2, 9.3).

It is important to give patients home exercises to improve the self-management of their musculoskeletal condition. Balance training is very simple to use and requires very little, if any, equipment so it is ideal for self-care.

Regular attendance at tai chi classes/practice will help achieve similar enhanced balance and stability.

The list below highlights some of the key background features that may require attention, or at least awareness.

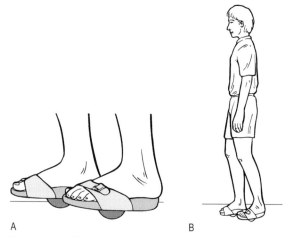

A   B

Figure 9.3   (A) Balance sandals to assist retraining (available from OPTP (800) 367 7393 USA). (B) Walking on balance sandals. (From Chaitow 2003.)

Possible soft-tissue and joint stressors contributing to back pain:

- Congenital factors, such as short leg, small hemipelvis
- Birth injury, such as cranial trauma from forceps delivery, distorts the internal cranial fascia – tentorium cerebelli and falx cerebri. Because of body-wide fascial continuity, this can cause distortions elsewhere

- Overuse, misuse, or abuse of the musculoskeletal system in work, recreational settings or close environment (chairs, shoes, car seat, etc.)
- Habitual postural stress
- Habitual upper chest breathing pattern
- Trauma: either repetitive minor forms or major incidents
- Reflexive factors, including myofascial trigger points and viscerosomatic influences
- Chronic somatization influences generated by negative psychological and emotional factors and coping traits, including fear, anger, anxiety, depression, etc.
- Biochemical changes resulting from nutritional, toxic, endocrine, infectious and other influences.

With some of the listed ingredients (above) interacting with the unique attributes of the individual, it should be possible to recognize an evolution towards dysfunction as outlined below. If so, the functional and structural changes that are palpable, visible or recognizable through clinical assessment, should be addressed using appropriate manual and movement methods.

The formula to remember is:

- Reduce the adaptive load (reduce or stop doing those things that are adding to compensatory processes: better posture, better use patterns, better breathing, etc.)
- Improve function (mobilize, strengthen, loosen – as appropriate – allowing better handling of adaptive load).

Once these aspects are being addressed, self-regulation (homeostasis) ensures that improvement should follow.

PROGRESSIVE ADAPTIVE CHANGES TO SOFT TISSUE STRESSORS

Progressive adaptive changes to soft tissue stressors (Digiovanna 1991, Greenman 1996, Janda 1982, Liebenson 1995) are as follows:

1 When tissues are stressed an initial 'alarm' response occurs in which tissues become hypertonic and/or painful
2 If such changes are other than short term, localized oxygen deficit is probable, together with retention of metabolic waste products, both of which result in discomfort or pain and the likelihood of an increased hypertonic response
3 The constant activity of the neural reporting stations in these tissues leads to increased neural sensitization and the development of a tendency to hyperreactivity (known in osteopathic medicine as 'facilitation')

4 Macrophages become activated – along with increased vascularity, fibroblast action and connective tissue production – leading to cross-linkage and shortening of tissues
5 Changes take place in the muscles as a result of hypertonicity which, if sustained, lead to progressive fibrotic modification
6 Sustained hypertonicity produces drag on tendinous attachment to the periosteum and the likelihood of (periosteal) pain and dysfunction in these tissues
7 If such stressed tendons or muscles cross joints, they become crowded and their function is modified
8 The antagonists of chronically hypertonic muscles are reciprocally inhibited; as a result, normal firing sequences of muscles may alter, e.g. excessive activity of synergist muscles occurs in order to take on the tasks of weakened (inhibited) prime movers, or synergists
9 Chronically shortened hypertonic structures have a sustained inhibitory effect on their antagonists
10 One example is the short, tight, erector spinae muscles and weakened (inhibited) abdominal muscles seen in the typical 'slouching,' pot-bellied, sway-back posture ('crossed syndrome', see below)
11 Another example is the inhibition of deep neck flexors associated with short tight neck extensor muscles, seen in the typical 'chin-poke' head position
12 Posture, breathing and general function becomes less efficient, and energy is wasted in maintaining unnatural levels of tone, with fatigue a natural result.

UPPER AND LOWER CROSSED SYNDROMES

See Chapter 4 for more on this topic, and also Figure 4.9.

- Chain reactions of these dysfunctional patterns can occur, resulting from the shortening over time of postural muscles (type 1 fibers) and the inhibition and weakening (without shortening) of phasic muscles (type 2 fibers)
- Localized areas of hyperreactivity (facilitation) may evolve paraspinally, or in particular stress-prone regions of any myofascial structures, involving trigger points and other reflexively related changes
- These triggers themselves commonly become sources of pain and of further dysfunction

- Postural and functional changes will become apparent throughout the body, e.g. in relation to breathing pattern dysfunction ('upper chest breathing'), which can result from (for example) poor, slumped posture, and which cannot be easily normalized until the structural changes that encourage it are corrected
- Therapeutic input in response to such changes must address the multiple changes that have occurred, to reduce hypertonicity, resolve fibrotic changes, lengthen shortened structures, tone weakened/ inhibited structures, mobilize joints, deactivate trigger points, as well as to remove habitual patterns of use that have added to or caused the dysfunctional patterns, including postural and respiratory re-education
- The musculoskeletal changes described previously may have biomechanical, biochemical, and psychological components, all of which must be understood and, if possible, modified or removed.

THE THERAPIST'S ROLE

Your role as a therapist is to advise the patient as to the best way(s) of modifying this downward spiral, with therapy as a means of modifying the effects, and to encourage more normal function ideally through homework/self-management.

Long-term prevention depends on stopping the behaviors that produced the problem in the first place, or on reducing the impact of features that cannot be removed (arthritic changes, unbalanced leg length, for example).

In this context, focus on stress management, sleep and exercise patterns and emotional well-being, all play a major part.

References

Bohannon R W, Larkin P A, Cook A C et al 1984 Decrease in timed balance test scores with aging. Physical Therapy 64(7):1067–1070

Chaitow L 2003 Maintaining body balance, flexibility and stability. Churchill Livingstone, Edinburgh

DiGiovanna E (ed.) 1991 An osteopathic approach to diagnosis and treatment. Lippincott, Philadelphia

Greenman P 1996 Principles of manual medicine. Williams & Wilkins, Baltimore

Janda V 1982 Introduction to functional pathology of the motor system. Proceedings of the VIIth Commonwealth and International Conference on Sport. Physiotherapy and Sport 3:39

Janda V 1984 Low back pain: Trends, controversies, community-based rehabilitation approach. In: Proceedings from the Consultation on Disability Prevention and Rehabilitation, Turku, Finland

Liebenson C S 1995 Rehabilitation of the spine. Williams & Wilkins, Baltimore

Liebenson C S 2001 Advice for clinician and patient: Sensory-motor training. Journal for Bodywork and Movement Therapies 5(1):21–28

Chapter **10**

Other methods

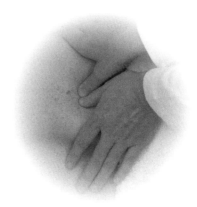

SUMMARY OF SYSTEMS, METHODS AND MODALITIES USED IN THE MANUAL TREATMENT OF BACK PAIN

There is an inevitable overlap in this attempt to summarize and define different, yet similar, approaches to the treatment and rehabilitation of back pain. Many of the systems have borrowed extensively from each other, and with 'evidence based' medicine now so widespread, it is becoming clear that the traditional differences between systems such as osteopathy and chiropractic, as examples, is narrowing. At the same time, an eclectic selection of methods and modalities is entering physical therapy and physiatry, to the extent that in some settings it is no longer possible to distinguish, from what is being done therapeutically, to which profession a practitioner belongs. This brief summary is not comprehensive, but hopefully offers an overview of what is available. Referral to other therapists and practitioners is strongly advised whenever areas of the patient's dysfunctional pattern seem to be outside your area of competence.

Massage therapy can be usefully combined with almost all of the methods and systems listed in Tables 10.1 and 10.2.

Table 10.1 Systems and methods

System	Abbreviated description
Osteopathy	In the USA, osteopathy is a primary care system that couples mainstream medical care with manipulation aimed at enhancing biomechanical, neurological, circulatory and other functions of the body. In the rest of the world, osteopathy is largely regulated, but has a more limited musculoskeletal focus with DOs focusing on what they term 'somatic dysfunction'. Many of the soft tissue methods discussed in this text (MET, PRT for example) evolved out of osteopathic methodology.
Chiropractic	Chiropractic uses manipulative and rehabilitation methods to normalize restricted joint function (subluxations) using, as a main tool, high velocity thrust adjustments. Increasingly DCs are using other, less invasive approaches.
Physical therapy	PTs have traditionally been seen as a profession supplementary to medicine, but are increasingly becoming first line practitioners, focusing largely on rehabilitation (post-surgery, post-trauma, etc.). PTs now use many of the methods developed by DCs and DOs; who in turn are increasingly using the rehabilitation methods developed in physical therapy.
Exercise rehabilitation	A wide range of variably trained practitioners and therapists use exercises in prevention, treatment and rehabilitation contexts; aimed at specific joints or general posture, for example. The best known methods, such as the Alexander Technique, Athletic training, Pilates and Feldenkrais, have a large educational component, with some focusing on core stability and others on enhanced use of the body.
Massage	Massage therapy is gradually dividing into broad categories which focus on either 'wellness/relaxation', or therapeutic intervention (often in athletic contexts), with many LMTs also incorporating rehabilitation exercise methods. Standards vary worldwide from excellent to poor, with major efforts underway to raise training standards, as research validates the importance of this traditional approach to health and healing. A number of ethnic variations such as Ayurvedic and Thai massage are becoming increasingly researched and used.
Prolotherapy	An increasingly commonly used approach aimed at creating repetitive irritation of connective tissue (using various injected substances) to help normalize unstable joints such as sacroiliac.
TCM (in addition to acupuncture)	Tuina methods used in TCM have many of the characteristics of osteopathy and chiropractic as well as a range of unique soft tissue methods.
Soft tissue manipulation	See Table 10.2.
Physiatry	A branch of medicine that utilizes an eclectic selection of manipulation and other methods (e.g. prolotherapy) in treatment of musculoskeletal dysfunction.
Movement therapy	Yoga, Tai chi, Chi Gung, Trager work, Aston patterning, etc. are examples of this large area of care which enjoys increasing respect as the methods are validated by research, in both therapeutic and rehabilitation settings.

MET, muscle energy technique; PRT, positional release technique; PTs, physical therapists; DOs, osteopaths; DCs, chiropractors; LMTs, licensed massage therapists; TCM, traditional Chinese Medicine.

Table 10.2 Soft tissue manipulation methods

Technique	Description
Articulation	Repetitive passive movements employing leverage through variable ranges of the arc.
Effleurage	Superficial drainage technique derived from massage therapy.
Inhibition/ischemic compression	Describes an objective rather than a method; consists of pressure applied for lengthy periods, slowly applied and slowly released, using thumb contact as a rule.
Kneading	Deep or superficial rhythmical pressure, usually applied by thenar or hypothenar eminence.
Positional release techniques (PRT)	Approaches that, instead of acting directly on restricted or shortened structures, aim to position them in a state of 'ease' by moving away from restriction barriers, allowing a spontaneous normalization to occur, involving neural (muscle spindle) resetting and circulatory enhancement. These methods include what is known as strain/counterstrain, as well as much craniosacral work.
Rhythmic traction	Repetitive attempts to separate articulations in order to stretch interarticular and periarticular structures.
Springing	Repetitive, usually slowly applied, pressure of a gradual nature, often used diagnostically.
Stretching	Short and long amplitude attempts at separation of muscular attachments, and stretch of ligaments, fascia, and membranes.
Vibration	Rapid oscillatory pressure or movement.
Muscle energy techniques (MET)	Use of variations on the theme of isometric and isotonic contractions to initiate increased tolerance to stretching of shortened muscle, and/or increased tone (facilitation) of inhibited muscles.
Neuromuscular techniques (NMT)	Integrated combinations of the methods listed above, together with unique assessment and treatment methods that 'meet and match' tissue tension – based originally on Ayurvedic massage.

Glossary

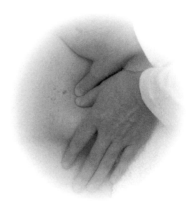

Active joint movement Movement of a joint by the patient/client, in contrast to *passive joint movement*, in which all motion is produced by the therapist.

Adaptation The process whereby the person or the area responds to physical, chemical or psychosocial demands. E.g. Muscles adapt to regular exercise by gaining in bulk and strength; while the person as a whole adapts to exercise by gaining aerobic fitness.

Adherence Used in the context of whether a patient/client 'adheres' to ('sticks to, or follows) the advice given by a therapist/practitioner. Previously described as 'compliance', and more recently called by some 'concordance'.

Alexander technique A postural re-education system

Algometer A pressure gauge used to measure amount of force being applied during treatment of, say, trigger points.

Amplitude In the context of manipulation how the distance over which an adjustment's force is applied. HVLA – High velocity (very rapid), low amplitude (short distance) is the way chiropractic and osteopathic manipulation is described.

Ankylosing spondylitis An autoimmune disease, mainly affecting males, that leads to a gradual fusion of the spine and pelvic joints, resulting in the individual being locked into a very stooped posture ('bamboo spine').

Antagonist The opposite muscle to one that is active (known as the agonist). E.g. the flexor muscles of the arm are the antagonists of the extensor muscles of the arm.

Anterior oblique muscle system Muscles that run obliquely across the abdomen forming part of the core stabilizing muscles.

Anti-arousal breathing A slow rhythmical breathing pattern (similar to pranayama yoga breathing) in which exhalation lasts at least twice as long as inhalation, and which reduces sympathetic arousal.

Articulation A joint is an articulation. The word articulation can also be used to describe a mobilizing approach that moves a joint through its full range of motion.

ARTT acronym ARTT stands for Asymmetry, Range of motion restriction, Tenderness, Tissue texture change.

ASIS (anterior superior iliac spine) The prominence on the front of the pelvis that is frequently used as a landmark during palpation.

Aston patterning A system of postural and self-use methods, devised by Judith Aston.

Asymmetry Unequal from side to side; left side different from right side.

Attachment point A trigger or tender point close to a tendon or site of periosteal attachment.

Ayurvedic (Indian) massage Traditional Indian methods deriving from Ayurvedic methods of treatment.

Balance training Learning to enhance the ability to balance by means of specific exercises.

'Beach pose' A position used in breathing retraining to stabilize shoulder movement on inhalation, in which the hands are interlocked behind the neck - as in the position often seen when lying on a beach sun-bathing.

Bending loading (force) The forces generated in specific tissues during bending.

'Bind' A shorthand term (the opposite of 'ease') describing tension, increased or unnatural levels of tone, or restriction.

'Blockage' A shorthand term describing a restricted range of motion in a joint.

Breathing wave assessment Evaluation of the response/movement of the spine to deep inhalation when lying prone on a firm surface.

Brügger's relief position A particular sequence applied by the seated individual to enhance posture and function during performance of breathing exercises.

Catastrophizing Fearing the worst will happen; imagining that disaster lies just around the corner.

Cat–camel exercise An exercise performed on all fours in which the spine is sequentially flexed and extended (in part replicating a cat's stretching movements).

Catecholamine Any of various amines (as epinephrine, norepinephrine, and dopamine) that are derived from tyrosine, and that function as hormones or neurotransmitters or both.

Cauda equina syndrome A condition involving the roots of the upper sacral nerves that extend beyond the termination of the spinal cord at the first lumbar vertebra in the form of a bundle of filaments within the vertebral canal resembling a horse's tail.

Central point A trigger point that lies close to the motor end-point, near the belly of a muscle.

Centrifugal direction Spinning or rotating towards the centre.

Centripetal direction Spinning or rotating away from the centre.

Chakra Concept of energy centres deriving from Ayurvedic (Indian) traditional medicine.

Chi Gung An ancient Chinese martial art system, often used in the West for assisting postural and breathing functions. (Note: it has similarities to Tai Chi.)

'Chin-poke' head position A posture in which the head is held forward of its ideal position with the chin poked forward.

Cognitive behavior therapy (CBT) CBT is an interactive, directive approach that aims to help people who are ill or disabled to confront thoughts, beliefs and behaviors associated with their health.

Colloidal matrix Colloidal material in intercellular tissues.

Combined loading (force) A combination of forces applied to an area, for example shear force as well as compression.

Comfort zone A place, time or position where distress is minimized.

Compensation The consequence of an adaptation response. For example if there is pain when placing weight on the right foot a compensation will occur in which weight is transferred elsewhere in order to reduce discomfort.

Compression fracture A fracture that results from a compression (crushing) force.

Compression (compressive) loading (force) A force that crowds tissues, as in application of pressure by a hand or thumb.

Connective tissue massage A German manual system that uses strong finger or thumb strokes in order to elicit a reflex response.

Core stability (exercises) Exercises (such as Pilates) that aim to produce a balanced degree of tone, strength and stamina to the core muscles of the trunk (for example abdomen, low back, diaphragm).

Cortisol A hormone produced in response to stress.

Counterirritation For example briskly rubbing a painful area produces sensations that help to mask the pain, and this is a counter-irritation.

Crohn's disease An auto-immune inflammatory bowel disease.

Crossed syndrome Patterns of weak and tight muscles identified as alternating across the body – for example weak gluteals and tight psoas; or weak deep neck flexors and tight cervical erector spinae muscles.

Cystitis An irritation or inflammation of the bladder leading to feelings of urgency to urinate, and sometimes to burning discomfort on doing so.

'Dead-bug' exercise (test) A position in which a test of the strength/stamina of particular (core) muscles can be carried out, or in which strengthening exercises can be performed, that is reminiscent of a dead insect because the person lies on their back with legs and arms in the air.

Deconditioning When someone is out of condition, specifically when someone has not been performing aerobic activity.

Deep longitudinal muscle system Muscles that run in line with the body as opposed to muscles which run in different directions (e.g. obliques), and which are not superficial, i.e. they are deep.

Deep tissue massage Massage that addresses deeper soft tissue structures rather than superficial ones.

Depression A state of feeling sad; a psychoneurotic or psychotic disorder marked especially by sadness, inactivity, difficulty with thinking and concentration, a significant increase or decrease in appetite and time spent sleeping, feelings of dejection and hopelessness, and sometimes suicidal thoughts or an attempt to commit suicide.

Displacement The act or process of removing something from its usual or proper place or the state resulting from this.

Distress Pain or suffering affecting the body, a bodily part, or the mind, e.g. gastric distress.

Drag palpation assessment Use of a light finger stroke across tissues seeking a sensation of 'drag' created by increased water content (sweat) presumed to result from increased sympathetic activity in deeper tissues.

Duration The length of time something takes to occur.

Dysmenorrhea Painful menstruation.

Effleurage A light stroking movement used in massage.

Elastic limit (barrier) The limit, barrier, end-of-range to which tissues can be taken without damage.

Elasticity The quality or state of being elastic.

Embryonic point The early stages of development of a new trigger point.

'End feel' The palpated sense of the quality of resistance as a joint or muscle comes to its end of range – for example a 'soft end-feel' in a normal joint, or a 'hard end-feel' in a dysfunctional or degenerated joint.

Endorphin Any of a group of self-produced hormones (such as enkephalin) found especially in the brain that bind chiefly to opiate receptors and produce some of the same pharmacological effects (as pain relief) as those of opiates.

'Facilitation'
1. The lowering of the threshold for reflex conduction along a particular neural pathway especially from repeated use of that pathway.
2. The increasing of the ease or intensity of a response by repeated stimulation; the act or process of stimulating.

False negative Relating to or being an individual or a test result that is wrongly classified in a negative category because of imperfect testing methods or procedures.

False positive Relating to or being an individual or a test result that is wrongly classified in a positive category (as of diagnosis) because of imperfect testing methods or procedures (example: a *false-positive* pregnancy test).

Fasciculation Muscular twitching involving the simultaneous contraction of contiguous groups of muscle fibers.

Feldenkrais Used for a system of aided body movements intended to increase bodily awareness and ease tension.

Fibromyalgia A chronic disorder characterized by widespread pain, tenderness, and stiffness of muscles and associated connective tissue structures that is typically accompanied by fatigue, headache, and sleep disturbances.

Fibrosis A condition marked by increase of interstitial fibrous tissue; fibrous degeneration.

Filum terminale The slender threadlike prolongation of the spinal cord below the origin of the lumbar nerves; the last portion of the pia mater.

Fine-tuning A shorthand term for perfecting the positioning of a joint or area when identifying the maximum point of comfort, or ease.

Flare dysfunction Describes the positioning of the ilia in relation to the sacrum when a flaring outwards (lateral), or inwards (medial) occurs.

Force closure The influence of muscular forces in stabilization of the sacroiliac joint.

Form closure The influence of joint surfaces' (sacrum and ilium) forces to stabilize the sacroiliac joint.

Frequency How often something occurs.

Friction The effect of two or more surfaces rubbing together to produce mechanically induced heat and possibly inflammation.

GABA Abbreviation for gamma-aminobutyric acid: an amino acid that is a neurotransmitter that induces neural inhibition.

Gait cycle Gait describes a manner of walking or moving on foot – and the gait cycle describes the complete cycle of activity during the activity of gait when walking.

General adaptation syndromes (GAS) A theory that describes the stages of adaptation ranging from initial alarm, through adaptation, to exhaustion and collapse.

Golgi tendon organ A spindle-shaped sensory end organ within a tendon that provides information about muscle tension – called also *neurotendinous spindle.*

Grieve's masqueraders A series of symptoms described by Grieve that mimic simple conditions but which are in fact the result of serious pathology.

'Growing pain' A phrase used to describe pain experienced by a young person that is not easily identified or explained.

Guarding Involuntary reaction to protect an area of pain (as by spasm of muscle on palpation of the abdomen over a painful lesion).

Heel strike The moment of the grounding of the heel during a forward step in the gait cycle.

Hip abduction (observation) test A side-lying test that evaluates the firing sequence of muscles during hip abduction.

Hip extension test A prone test that evaluates the firing sequence of muscles during hip extension.

Homeostasis The maintenance of relatively stable internal physiological conditions (as body temperature) in higher animals under fluctuating environmental conditions.

Hydrosis Increased presence of water in tissues as in perspiration/sweat.

'Hyperalgesic skin zone' An area characterized by increased sensitivity to pain or enhanced intensity of pain sensation.

Hypermobility (laxness) An increase in the range of movement of which a bodily part and especially a joint is capable, commonly due to the looseness of ligaments.

Hyperreactivity Having or showing abnormally high sensitivity to stimuli – for example cystic fibrosis involves *hyperreactive* airways.

Hyperstimulation analgesia Excessive stimulation of an organ or part (e.g. nerve) leading to relief of pain without loss of consciousness.

Hypertonicity The quality or state of being hypertonic (having increased tone).

Hyperventilation Excessive ventilation; *specifically*: excessive rate and depth of respiration leading to abnormal loss of carbon dioxide from the blood – called also *overventilation*.

Iliosacral test, see Standing flexion (iliosacral) test Testing the functionality of the iliosacral joints during standing flexion.

Illness behavior Altered functionality resulting from a reaction to symptoms that is inappropriate. Commonly occurs when 'hurt' is translated as 'harm', when in fact no harm would arise from performing normal actions even though they hurt.

Imposter (masquerader) back pain (symptoms) Symptoms that result from more serious conditions/ pathology that mimic 'normal' back pain.

'Increased tolerance to stretch' (ITS) The effect that allows more force to be painlessly used in stretching, resulting from the use of isometric contractions in use of methods such as Muscle Energy Technique and PNF.

Inflammation A local response to cellular injury that is marked by capillary dilatation, leukocytic infiltration, redness, heat, pain, swelling, and often loss of function, and that serves as a mechanism initiating the elimination of noxious agents and of damaged tissue.

Inflare When an ilium flares medially in relation to the sacrum as part of a sacroiliac or iliosacral dysfunction.

Inhibition (ischemic compression) Interference with or retardation or prevention of a process or activity.

Integrated neuromuscular inhibition (INIT) An integrated sequence employed in trigger point deactivation.

Ischemic compression see Inhibition.

Isometric contraction A contraction where resistance to the effort is complete so that no movement occurs.

'Jump sign' A term used in relation to palpation and treatment of trigger points describing an inadvertent 'jump' when the trigger point is pressed.

Kneading (see Petrissage) Massage in which the muscles are kneaded.

Kyphosis Exaggerated outward curvature of the thoracic region of the spinal column resulting in a rounded upper back.

Landmark A feature of the body that can be observed or palpated.

Lateral muscle system Muscle groups that lie laterally rather than medially.

Laxness see Hypermobility.

Load, loading The application of pressure to tissues in one form or another, for example compressive or shearing.

Local adaptation syndromes (LAS) The same sequence that occurs in the General Adaptation Syndrome, but applied to a local area – for example a shoulder or knee being subjected to repetitive stresses.

Lomi Lomi massage A form of Hawaiian massage.

Lumbar zygapophysial (facet) syndrome A dysfunctional state of vertebral facet joints in the lumbar region.

Lumbodorsal fascia The wide band of fascia that links the lumbar spinal region to the pelvic and lower limb fascia (below) and thoracic and cervical fascia (above).

Lymphatic drainage methods Techniques that encourage enhanced lymphatic flow and drainage.

Masquerader symptoms see Imposter symptoms.

McGill Pain Questionnaire A specialized questionnaire that helps determine the degree and nature of pain being experienced.

Meridian Any of the pathways along which the body's vital energy flows according to the theory of acupuncture.

Microtrauma injury A very slight injury or lesion.

Mind–body techniques Methods that attempt to understand and treat somatic and emotional issues that are linked by trauma.

Morton's syndrome A form of metatarsalgia involving compression of a branch of the plantar nerve.

Movement therapy Treatment and rehabilitation methods involving active participation of the patient.

Muscle energy techniques (MET) Use of carefully modulated isometric and isotonic contractions to enhance mobility and length of dysfunctional tissues, developed as part of osteopathic medicine.

Muscle fatigue The temporary loss of power to respond induced in a sensory receptor or motor end organ by continued stimulation.

Muscle knot An area of unnatural tension or fibrosis in a muscle.

Muscle shortness tests Tests to evaluate normal length of muscles.

Muscle spindle A sensory end organ in a muscle that is sensitive to stretch in the muscle, consists of small striated muscle fibers richly supplied with nerve fibers, and is enclosed in a connective tissue sheath – called also *stretch receptor*.

Muscle weakness tests Tests to evaluate normal strength of muscles.

Myofascial release (MFR) A form of treatment that encourages increased length of the myofascial tissues by application of load in two directions simultaneously.

Nerve root compression Pressure on a nerve root, for example as a result of disc herniation.

Neuromuscular techniques (NMT) A series of manual treatment methods that use the effects of specific pressure and stretch approaches on the nervous system and myofascial tissues. There is a British (Lief's) NMT as well as an American version derived from the work of Nimmo.

Neuroresponse The response of the nervous system to a stimulus.

Nociceptor A receptor for injurious or painful stimuli; a pain sense organ.

Nodal point Either of two points so located on the axis of a lens or optical system that any incident ray directed through one will produce a parallel emergent ray directed through the other.

Operant conditioning Conditioning in which the desired behavior or increasingly closer approximations to it are followed by a rewarding or reinforcing stimulus.

Oscillation The action or state of oscillating (rhythmically or harmonically vibrating).

Osteitis deformans (Paget's disease) A chronic disease of bones characterized by their great enlargement and rarefaction with bowing of the long bones and deformation of the flat bones.

Osteopathy A system of medical practice based on a theory that diseases are due chiefly to loss of structural integrity which can be restored by manipulation of the parts supplemented by therapeutic measures (such as use of medicine or surgery).

Osteoporosis A condition that affects especially older women and is characterized by decrease in bone mass with decreased density and enlargement of bone spaces producing porosity and brittleness.

Outcome based massage Massage methodology based on anticipated outcome.

Outflare When an ilium flares laterally in relation to the sacrum as part of a sacroiliac or iliosacral dysfunction.

Paget's disease see Osteitis deformans.

'Pain behavior' see Illness behavior.

Pain drawing A sketch made by a patient of his/her pain.

Pain threshold The level of pressure or irritation required to trigger a sense of pain in the patient is the threshold.

Passive joint movement Movement produced by the practitioner without help from the patient.

Percussion Massage consisting of the striking of a body part with light rapid blows – called also *tapotement.*

Petrissage (kneading) see Kneading.

Physiatry The practice of physical medicine and rehabilitation.

Physical therapy The treatment of disease by physical and mechanical means (such as massage, regulated exercise, water, light, heat, and electricity) – called also *physiotherapy.*

Pilates Used for an exercise regimen typically performed with the use of specialized apparatus and designed to improve the overall condition of the body.

Pliability Being supple and flexible.

Positional release technique (PRT) Treatment methods that allow spontaneous improvement of dysfunctional tissues by placing them in a degree of supported comfort or 'ease' and either holding them there or taping them into an unloaded position.

Post-isometric relaxation (PIR) A response of tissues to be held in an isometric contraction.

Prolotherapy An alternative therapy for treating musculoskeletal pain that involves injecting an irritant substance (such as dextrose) into a ligament or tendon to promote the growth of new tissue.

Prone hip extension test see Hip extension test.

Prone trunk extension test see Trunk extension test.

Proprioception The reception of stimuli produced within the organism.

'Pseudo-sciatica' referral pattern A painful pattern in the lower limb that mimics true sciatica but which derives from other sources, such as a trigger point.

PSIS (posterior superior iliac spine) A landmark at the medial end of the crest of the pelvis posteriorly.

Pulsed MET Use of repetitive mini-isometric contractions against a restriction barrier to achieve a release.

Pursed lip breathing In breathing rehabilitation, exhaling slowly through a narrowed aperture created by pursing the lips as though blowing through a drinking straw.

Radicular pain Relating to, or involving a nerve root.

Range of motion The normal physiological range of motion of a joint or muscle.

Reciprocal inhibition (RI) The neurological effect affecting a muscle after its antagonist has been isometrically contracted.

Red (yellow) flags Red flags are signs or symptoms that suggest that a serious pathological condition exists. Yellow flags are signs or symptoms that suggest that psychosocial factors exist that increase the risk of developing, or perpetuating chronic pain and long-term disability.

Reflex activity An automatic and often inborn response to a stimulus that involves a nerve impulse passing inward from a receptor to the spinal cord and thence outward to an effector (such as a muscle or gland) without reaching the level of consciousness and often without passing to the brain, for example the knee-jerk *reflex*.

Reflexology A form of treatment based on the belief that reflex areas exist in the hands and feet (for example) which when compressed or rubbed, influence functions and systems distant from the area being treated.

Rehabilitation exercises Exercises used during the physical restoration of a sick or disabled person by therapeutic measures and re-education to participation in the activities of a normal life.

Restriction barrier The point beyond which easy, free, movement is not possible.

Rhythmic traction Repetitive traction performed in a rhythmic manner.

Rotation (torsion) loading (force) Application of load using a twisting (rotational) action.

Rotational dysfunction A dysfunctional situation either caused by a rotational movement, or preventing a rotational movement.

Scoliosis A lateral curvature of the spine.

Seated flexion (sacroiliac) test A flexion test performed with the patient seated to assess the presence of a restriction in the SI joint.

Serotonin An important neurotransmitter that is a powerful vasoconstrictor and is found especially in the brain, blood serum, and gastric mucous membrane of mammals.

Shear loading (shearing force) A loading force that creates a shearing pattern of strain in tissues.

Shiatsu Acupressure especially of a form that originated in Japan.

Side bridge exercise An exercise that assists in creating core stability in which the patient lies on his/her side and creates demands for support from lateral muscle groups.

Sliding force A loading force that causes one tissue to slide on another (for example skin on fascia).

Spondylolisthesis Forward displacement of a lumbar vertebra on the one below it and especially of the fifth lumbar vertebra on the sacrum producing pain by compression of nerve roots.

Standing flexion (iliosacral) test Testing the functionality of the iliosacral joints during standing flexion.

Stenosis A narrowing or constriction of the diameter of a bodily passage or orifice.

Strain/counterstrain (SCS) A positional release method.

Stress

1. A force exerted when one body or body part presses on, pulls on, pushes against, or tends to compress or twist another body or body part; *especially*: the intensity of this mutual force commonly expressed in pounds per square inch. The deformation caused in a body by such a force.

2. A physical, chemical, or emotional factor that causes bodily or mental tension and may be a factor in disease causation. A state of bodily or mental tension resulting from factors that tend to alter an existent equilibrium.

Subluxation Partial dislocation (such as of one of the bones in a joint). Used in chiropractic to describe an area of restriction/dysfunction.

Substance P A neuropeptide that consists of 11 amino acid residues, that is widely distributed in the brain, spinal cord, and peripheral nervous system, and that acts across nerve synapses to produce prolonged postsynaptic excitation.

Synergism Interaction of discrete agents such that the total effect is greater than the sum of the individual effects – such as a group of muscles working together.

Tai chi An ancient Chinese discipline involving a continuous series of controlled, usually slow movements designed to improve physical and mental well-being – called also *t'ai chi ch'uan, tai chi chuan*.

Tapotement Percussion during massage.

Taut band A localized area of tissue tightness associated with trigger points.

'Tender' point An area that is more tender to pressure than is appropriate (i.e. where pain threshold has lowered).

Tension (tensile) loading (force) A loading force that creates tension in the tissues being treated.

Tissue texture What tissue feels like to the therapist when palpated (fibrous, swollen, loose etc.).

Toe-off The moment that the foot leaves contact with the surface during the gait cycle.

Tone Normal tissue tension or responsiveness to stimuli.

Torsion The state of being twisted.

Transcutaneous electrical stimulation Passage of an electrical current across painful tissues to produce pain relief.

Triage The sorting of patients according to the urgency of their need for care.

Trunk extension test A test to evaluate strength of the multifidi in which the prone patient extends the spine while ensuring legs and feet remain in contact with the floor at all times. Failure to do so suggests weakness.

Tuina methods Traditional Chinese Medicine massage and manipulation methods.

Type I muscle fibers Fibers that have a primarily supportive/postural function in muscles.

Type II muscle fibers Fibers that have a primarily phasic/movement function in muscles.

Vapocoolant spray A spray that cools tissues.

Visceral drag The effect of sagging organs as in visceroptosis.

Visceroptosis Downward displacement of the abdominal organs.

Visual analog scale (VAS) A tool (line on a piece of paper) on which the degree of pain being experienced can be recorded by the patient.

Index

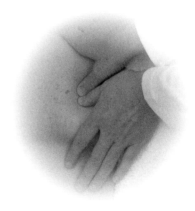

ELSEVIER DVD-ROM LICENCE AGREEMENT

PLEASE READ THE FOLLOWING AGREEMENT CAREFULLY BEFORE USING THIS PRODUCT. THIS PRODUCT IS LICENSED UNDER THE TERMS CONTAINED IN THIS LICENCE AGREEMENT ("Agreement"). BY USING THIS PRODUCT, YOU, AN INDIVIDUAL OR ENTITY INCLUDING EMPLOYEES, AGENTS AND REPRESENTATIVES ("You" or "Your"), ACKNOWLEDGE THAT YOU HAVE READ THIS AGREEMENT, THAT YOU UNDERSTAND IT, AND THAT YOU AGREE TO BE BOUND BY THE TERMS AND CONDITIONS OF THIS AGREEMENT. ELSEVIER LIMITED ("Elsevier") EXPRESSLY DOES NOT AGREE TO LICENSE THIS PRODUCT TO YOU UNLESS YOU ASSENT TO THIS AGREEMENT. IF YOU DO NOT AGREE WITH ANY OF THE FOLLOWING TERMS, YOU MAY, WITHIN THIRTY (30) DAYS AFTER YOUR RECEIPT OF THIS PRODUCT RETURN THE UNUSED PRODUCT AND ALL ACCOMPANYING DOCUMENTATION TO ELSEVIER FOR A FULL REFUND.

DEFINITIONS As used in this Agreement, these terms shall have the following meanings:

"Proprietary Material" means the valuable and proprietary information content of this Product including without limitation all indexes and graphic materials and software used to access, index, search and retrieve the information content from this Product developed or licensed by Elsevier and/or its affiliates, suppliers and licensors.

"Product" means the copy of the Proprietary Material and any other material delivered on DVD-ROM and any other human readable or machine-readable materials enclosed with this Agreement, including without limitation documentation relating to the same.

OWNERSHIP This Product has been supplied by and is proprietary to Elsevier and/or its affiliates, suppliers and licensors. The copyright in the Product belongs to Elsevier and/or its affiliates, suppliers and licensors and is protected by the copyright, trademark, trade secret and other intellectual property laws of the United Kingdom and international treaty provisions, including without limitation the Universal Copyright Convention and the Berne Copyright Convention. You have no ownership rights in this Product. Except as expressly set forth herein, no part of this Product, including without limitation the Proprietary Material, may be modified, copied or distributed in hardcopy or machine-readable form without prior written consent from Elsevier. All rights not expressly granted to You herein are expressly reserved. Any other use of this Product by any person or entity is strictly prohibited and a violation of this Agreement.

SCOPE OF RIGHTS LICENSED (PERMITTED USES) Elsevier is granting to You a limited, non-exclusive, non-transferable licence to use this Product in accordance with the terms of this Agreement. You may use or provide access to this Product on a single computer or terminal physically located at Your premises and in a secure network or move this Product to and use it on another single computer or terminal at the same location for personal use only, but under no circumstances may You use or provide access to any part or parts of this Product on more than one computer or terminal simultaneously.

You shall not (a) copy, download, or otherwise reproduce the Product or any part(s) thereof in any medium, including, without limitation, online transmissions, local area networks, wide area networks, intranets, extranets and the Internet, or in any way, in whole or in part, except for printing out or downloading nonsubstantial portions of the text and images in the Product for Your own personal use; (b) alter, modify, or adapt the Product or any part(s) thereof, including but not limited to decompiling, disassembling, reverse engineering, or creating derivative works, without the prior written approval of Elsevier; (c) sell, license or otherwise distribute to third parties the Product or any part(s) thereof; or (d) alter, remove, obscure or obstruct the display of any copyright, trademark or other proprietary notice on or in the Product or on any printout or download of portions of the Proprietary Materials.

RESTRICTIONS ON TRANSFER This Licence is personal to You, and neither Your rights hereunder nor the tangible embodiments of this Product, including without limitation the Proprietary Material, may be sold, assigned, transferred or sublicensed to any other person, including without limitation by operation of law, without the prior written consent of Elsevier. Any purported sale, assignment, transfer or sublicense without the prior written consent of Elsevier will be void and will automatically terminate the Licence granted hereunder.

TERM This Agreement will remain in effect until terminated pursuant to the terms of this Agreement. You may terminate this Agreement at any time by removing from Your system and destroying the Product and any copies of the Proprietary Material. Unauthorized copying of the Product, including without limitation, the Proprietary Material and documentation, or otherwise failing to comply with the terms and conditions of this Agreement shall result in automatic termination of this licence and will make available to Elsevier legal remedies. Upon termination of this Agreement, the licence granted herein will terminate and You must immediately destroy the

Product and all copies of the Product and of the Proprietary Material, together with any and all accompanying documentation. All provisions relating to proprietary rights shall survive termination of this Agreement.

LIMITED WARRANTY AND LIMITATION OF LIABILITY Elsevier warrants that the software embodied in this Product will perform in substantial compliance with the documentation supplied in this Product, unless the performance problems are the result of hardware failure or improper use. If You report a significant defect in performance in writing to Elsevier within ninety (90) calendar days of your having purchased the Product, and Elsevier is not able to correct same within sixty (60) days after its receipt of Your notification, You may return this Product, including all copies and documentation, to Elsevier and Elsevier will refund Your money. In order to apply for a refund on your purchased Product, please contact the return address on the invoice to obtain the refund request form ("Refund Request Form"), and either fax or mail your signed request and your proof of purchase to the address indicated on the Refund Request Form. Incomplete forms will not be processed. Defined terms in the Refund Request Form shall have the same meaning as in this Agreement.

YOU UNDERSTAND THAT, EXCEPT FOR THE LIMITED WARRANTY RECITED ABOVE, ELSEVIER, ITS AFFILIATES, LICENSORS, THIRD PARTY SUPPLIERS AND AGENTS (TOGETHER "THE SUPPLIERS") MAKE NO REPRESENTATIONS OR WARRANTIES, WITH RESPECT TO THE PRODUCT, INCLUDING, WITHOUT LIMITATION THE PRO-PRIETARY MATERIAL. ALL OTHER REPRESEN-TATIONS, WARRANTIES, CONDITIONS OR OTHER TERMS, WHETHER EXPRESS OR IMPLIED BY STATUTE OR COMMON LAW, ARE HEREBY EXCLUDED TO THE FULLEST EXTENT PERMITTED BY LAW.

IN PARTICULAR BUT WITHOUT LIMITATION TO THE FOREGOING NONE OF THE SUPPLIERS MAKE ANY REPRESENTATIONS OR WARRANTIES (WHETHER EXPRESS OR IMPLIED) REGARDING THE PERFORMANCE OF YOUR PAD, NETWORK OR COMPUTER SYSTEM WHEN USED IN CON-JUNCTION WITH THE PRODUCT, NOR THAT THE PRODUCT WILL MEET YOUR REQUIREMENTS OR THAT ITS OPERATION WILL BE UNINTERRUPTED OR ERROR-FREE.

EXCEPT IN RESPECT OF DEATH OR PERSONAL INJURY CAUSED BY THE SUPPLIERS' NEGLIGENCE AND TO THE FULLEST EXTENT PERMITTED BY LAW, IN NO EVENT (AND REGARDLESS OF WHETHER SUCH DAMAGES ARE FORESEEABLE AND OF WHETHER SUCH LIABILITY IS BASED IN TORT, CONTRACT OR OTHERWISE) WILL ANY OF THE SUPPLIERS BE LIABLE TO YOU FOR ANY DAMAGES (INCLUDING, WITHOUT LIMITATION, ANY LOST PROFITS, LOST SAVINGS OR OTHER SPECIAL, INDIRECT, INCIDENTAL OR CONSE-QUENTIAL DAMAGES ARISING OUT OF OR RESULTING FROM: (I) YOUR USE OF, OR IN-ABILITY TO USE, THE PRODUCT; (II) DATA LOSS OR CORRUPTION; AND/OR (III) ERRORS OR OMISSIONS IN THE PROPRIETARY MATERIAL.

IF THE FOREGOING LIMITATION IS HELD TO BE UNENFORCEABLE, OUR MAXIMUM LIABILITY TO YOU IN RESPECT THEREOF SHALL NOT EXCEED THE AMOUNT OF THE LICENCE FEE PAID BY YOU FOR THE PRODUCT. THE REMEDIES AVAILABLE TO YOU AGAINST ELSEVIER AND THE LICENSORS OF MATERIALS INCLUDED IN THE PRODUCT ARE EXCLUSIVE.

If the information provided In the Product contains medical or health sciences information, it is intended for professional use within the medical field. Information about medical treatment or drug dosages is intended strictly for professional use, and because of rapid advances in the medical sciences, independent verification of diagnosis and drug dosages should be made. The provisions of this Agreement shall be severable, and in the event that any provision of this Agreement is found to be legally unenforceable, such unenforceability shall not prevent the enforcement or any other provision of this Agreement.

GOVERNING LAW This Agreement shall be governed by the laws of England and Wales. In any dispute arising out of this Agreement, you and Elsevier each consent to the exclusive personal jurisdiction and venue in the courts of England and Wales.

Minimum system requirements

Windows®
Windows 2000 or higher
Pentium® processor-based PC
128 MB RAM
4 X or faster DVD-ROM drive
VGA monitor supporting thousands of colours (16-bit)

Macintosh®
Apple Power Macintosh
Mac OS version 9 or later
128 MB of available RAM
4 X or faster DVD-ROM drive

NB: No data is transferred to the hard disk.
The DVD-ROM is self-contained and the application runs directly from the DVD-ROM.

Installation instructions

Windows®
If your system does not support Autorun, navigate to your DVD drive and double click on 'Start' to begin.

Alternatively, click Start, Run and type 'D:Start' to begin. If D: is not your DVD drive, substitute D: with the appropriate drive letter.

Macintosh®
If the DVD does not autorun, open the DVD icon that appears on the desktop and select 'Start' to begin.

To enable the DVD-ROM to autorun, select the Control Panels from the Apple menu on your desktop. Select QuickTime settings, then select Autoplay. Click the Enable DVD-ROM Autoplay checkbox, and then save the settings.

Using this Product
This product is designed to run with Internet Explorer 6.0 or later (PC) and Netscape 4.5 or later (Mac). Please refer to the help files on those programs for problems specific to the browser.

To use some of the functions on the DVD, the user must have the following:

a. DVD requires "Java Runtime Environment" to be installed in your system to use "Export" and "Slide Show" features. DVD automatically checks for "Java Runtime Environment" version 1.4.1 or later (PC) and MRJ 2.2.5 (Mac) if not available, it starts installing from the DVD. Please complete the installation process. Then click on the license agreement to proceed. "Java Runtime Environment" is available in the DVD's Software folder. If the user manually install the software, please make sure that the user start the application by clicking 'j2re-1_4_1_01-windows-i586.exe'.

b. Your browser needs to be Java-enabled. If the user did not enable Java when installing your browser, the user may need to download some additional files from your browser manufacturer.

c. If your system does not support Autorun, then please explore the DVD contents click on 'Start'.exe' to start.

d. QuickTime must be installed in order to view the video clips. A version of QuickTime is available in the DVD's Software folder.

Acrobat Reader can be installed from the Software folder of the DVD.

Viewing Images
You can view images by chapter and export images to PowerPoint or an HTML presentation. Full details are available in the Help section of the DVD-Rom.

Frequently Asked Questions (FAQ)

Do I need to have internet connection to run this program?

No. The program is designed to run entirely from the DVD-ROM, independent of the Internet. However the disk may contain some links to material on the Internet (website link) and to view this material you will require an Internet connection.

When I launch the application, I get messages after Netscape starts. What do I do?

TCP/IP is required to run any browserbased application. TCP/IP is included with Windows 95, 98 and NT. To add TCP/IP in Windows 95/98/NT, go to Network in the Control Panel. Click the Add button. Click the protocol option and click Add. Under manufacturers, select Microsoft and under Network Protrocols, select TCP/IP and click OK. Click OK again and Windows will start to install TCP/IP. When finished you will have to restart your machine.

What should I do if when I launch the application my ISP starts to dial out?

This application is able to run with or without a connection to the Internet. If your ISP starts to dial out, you can cancel this and the program will still run. Many ISPs will automatically dial out when a browser is launched. You may be able to turn this option off in the properties for your ISP.

When opening the DVD-ROM in Internet Explorer on the Mac my default home page opens. What should I do? When you run the DVD-ROM in Internet Explorer on the Mac two windows are opened – your default home page and the opening page of the DVD-ROM. Simply close the window that contains your default home page. We recommend, however, that Mac users view the DVD-ROM in Netscape.

The export function is not working properly. What should I do?

The Export feature requires the DVD-ROM Server to run in the background. The Server application requires the "Java Runtime Environment" to be installed in the system. The Server can be started manually by selecting 'server.exe' in Windows and 'server' application in MacOS.

Technical Support

Technical support for this product is available between 7.30 a.m. and 7.00 p.m. CST, Monday through Friday.

Before calling, be sure that your computer meets the minimum system requirements to run this software. Inside the United States and Canada, call 1-800-692-9010.
Inside the United Kingdom, call 00-800-692-90100.
Outside North America, call +1-314-872-8370.
You may also fax your questions to +1-314-997-5080, or contact Technical Support through e-mail: technical.support@elsevier.com.